# CHILDHOOD SPEECH AND LANGUAGE DISORDERS

# Whole Family Approaches to Childhood Illness and Disorders Series

Series Editor: Brian J. Fligor, ScD, board-certified audiologist and chief audiology officer at Lantos Technologies, Inc. brian.fligor@gmail.com

Whole Family Approaches to Childhood Illness and Disorders is a series of books authored by distinguished healthcare providers and developmental experts who focus on the whole family's experience when it comes to caring for a child with a particular health condition. Given that childhood illness and disability affects not just the child but also each member of the family, the care provided to the child must be done in the context of his family unit. Illness and disability in children occurs randomly, often without warning, and affects people of every race, religion, education, and economic status. When it happens, families are often in a state of chaos trying to negotiate multiple medical and therapy appointments, learning a whole new technical language around the condition, perhaps while grieving the diagnosis. Each book in this series serves as an opportunity for the author to share all of his or her wisdom with the reader, not just what can be covered in brief face-to-face meetings. Authors in this series provide important information about the condition, as well as pragmatic "how to navigate this situation," while validating the reader's emotions. It is the intent of this series to enlighten and support families as they blaze a trail to a new normal.

### Titles in the Series

*Understanding Childhood Hearing Loss: Whole Family Approaches to Living and Thriving*, by Brian J. Fligor

*Childhood Speech and Language Disorders: Supporting Children and Families on the Path to Communication*, by Suzanne M. Ducharme

# CHILDHOOD SPEECH AND LANGUAGE DISORDERS

## Supporting Children and Families on the Path to Communication

### Suzanne M. Ducharme

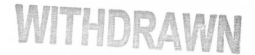

ROWMAN & LITTLEFIELD
Lanham • Boulder • New York • London

Published by Rowman & Littlefield
A wholly owned subsidiary of The Rowman & Littlefield Publishing Group, Inc.
4501 Forbes Boulevard, Suite 200, Lanham, Maryland 20706
www.rowman.com

Unit A, Whitacre Mews, 26-34 Stannary Street, London SE11 4AB

British Library Cataloguing in Publication Information Available

**Library of Congress Cataloging-in-Publication Data**

Names: Ducharme, Suzanne M., author.
Title: Childhood speech and language disorders : Supporting Children and Families on the Path to Communication / Suzanne M. Ducharme.
Description: Lanham : Rowman & Littlefield, [2016] | Series: Whole family approaches to childhood llness and disorders series | Includes bibliographical references and index.
Identifiers: LCCN 2016011434 (print) | LCCN 2016016869 (ebook) | ISBN 9781442238459 (cloth : alk. paper) | ISBN 9781442238466 (Electronic)
Subjects: LCSH: Speech disorders in children. | Language disorders in children. | Speech therapy for children.
Classification: LCC RJ496.S7 D83 2016 (print) | LCC RJ496.S7 (ebook) | DDC 618.92/855—dc23
LC record available at https://lccn.loc.gov/2016011434

♾ ™ The paper used in this publication meets the minimum requirements of American National Standard for Information Sciences Permanence of Paper for Printed Library Materials, ANSI/NISO Z39.48-1992.

Printed in the United States of America

# CONTENTS

# FOREWORD

As the father of four children, I have intimate knowledge of how a parent treasures his sons and daughters. They are more precious to me than anything else. There are no limits to what I would do to smooth their path in life, or limitations to what I would do to protect them from harm. My children are also relatively typical in their health and wellness: some food allergy issues, chronic ear infections, and a speech-language delay. As director of diagnostic audiology at Boston Children's Hospital, Boston, Massachusetts, from 2005 to 2013, I also have a great deal of experience with families of children who have health challenges: from milder, more easily treated health problems to severe, permanent disabilities that, in many ways, define the child's and family's life. This series, Whole Family Approaches to Childhood Illness and Disorders, will explore the many facets of childhood health and wellness and the problems that often, and randomly, occur and impact not just the child, but the immediate and extended family. Health care providers from many different disciplines are participating authors in this series. All share the perspective that they treat the child *and* the family, and not just the illness or developmental condition itself. These authors are among the most sophisticated clinicians in their respective fields but have also been invited to become authors in this series because they have unique empathy for children, parents, siblings, and extended family. In a very broad sense, the extended family does not have a clearly defined end point; perhaps a child has many blood relatives living in close proximity, but maybe that child's community is defined by membership in a religious institution, or that community may be defined by the historical shared experience of an entire ethnic group. The impact of childhood illness and disorders ripples throughout society, so a societal approach to treating children and their families with dignity and compassion requires a broad definition of "whole family."

Societies have struggled with how to balance the needs of the community with the needs of individuals, particularly in relation to to illnesses and disabilities, which have always been part of the human condition. Our human history doesn't have a very good track record related to the treatment of those who are ill or disabled. This is illustrated by the practice of abandonment of any infant not deemed healthy and strong by the Spartans of ancient Greece, or the murder of those with physical and mental disabilities by Nazi Germany in the 1940s. In the last half century, there has been a "Rights Revolution," which includes the protection of civil liberties of women, children, animals, racial and ethnic minorities, and those with illness or disability. In 1990, President George H. W. Bush signed into law the Americans with Disabilities Act (ADA), which prohibits discrimination and guarantees the civil rights of those with physical or mental disabilities. Modeled after the Civil Rights Act of 1964 (which prohibits discrimination based on race, color, religion, sex, or national origin), the ADA mandates that society provide equal access to employment, education, and participation in government programs and services for those with physical or mental disabilities. Rather than discard or hide away those with illness or disability, it is now considered culturally appropriate to include those with health or developmental challenges in all facets of society. In fact, it is incumbent on those of us without such challenges to ensure accessibility to our community institutions for those who would otherwise be excluded. To provide full inclusion in society of those with illness or disability elevates our own humanity and gives us every opportunity to benefit from the contributions of all members of society.

While he has been somewhat a reluctant advocate for civil rights of those with disabilities, Dr. Stephen Hawking serves as a wonderful example of the benefits to society when we make heroic efforts to provide access for all persons, regardless of health and wellness, to participate in society. Dr. Hawking is a renowned theoretical physicist, known most broadly for his work explaining the most basic laws governing the universe. His work has demonstrated a need to unify Einstein's general theory of relativity with quantum mechanics. Basically, he's one of the smartest people to ever populate the Earth. He also has a rare, early-onset form of amyotrophic lateral sclerosis (ALS, also known as Lou Gehrig's disease), which was diagnosed when he was twenty-one years old. The condition gradually progressed from his losing the ability to walk unassisted and his speech becoming slurred to his being unable to move or communicate without assistance. Dr. Hawking communicates using a computer-based communication system that is mounted on an arm on his wheelchair, and he uses the movement of his cheek to interface with this computer to type out messages to send to his speech synthesizer. Now at seventy-four years old, he is a prolific writer and lecturer and has received a fair amount of celebrity in popular media, including guest starring on the television show *The Big Bang Theory*. How many more Stephen Hawkings have there been in human history, whose talents have been lost because they either didn't survive or were disenfranchised (placed in an institution that provided care, but no opportunity for education and engagement)?

Communication is the key to a person's engagement with the rest of society. It is one of the most complicated things we do as humans, both physically (coordination of lips, tongue, vocal cords, and breath through very rapid movements) and cognitively (sending or receiving messages that are decoded in the brain). Given the sophistication of human communication, it should be no surprise that developing this system isn't always trivial. A multitude of children, every year, are found to be "late-talkers." Some of these late-talkers have underlying disorders that first show themselves as a speech delay: disorders such as autism, hearing loss, or selective language impairment. Identifying the underlying problem and establishing an appropriate intervention plan is squarely in the realm of the speech-language pathologist. In *Childhood Speech and Language Disorders: Supporting Children and Their Parents on the Path to Communication*, author and speech-language pathologist Suzanne Ducharme, MS, CCC-SLP, provides the reader with an easily understood, but in-depth, overview of speech and language in children: both typical as well as delayed or disordered communication development. This overview is most appropriate for decoding the "medical speak" parents may face when they are going through a myriad of appointments with specialists trying to figure out how best to support their child's communication development. Following this carefully constructed primer on speech and language disorders and therapeutic interventions, Ms. Ducharme gives equal time and attention to supporting parents in their journey with a child with a communication disorder. Whether the speech and/or language delay is in isolation, or one of a laundry list of challenges, *Childhood Speech and Language Disorders* can serve as validation of parents' emotions, a guidebook for getting organized, and a resource to become an effective advocate for care and education that is the child's right.

Ms. Ducharme has a wealth of experience as a speech-language pathologist: from supporting feeding and communication development in children being treated in the neonatal intensive care unit, to providing direct speech-language therapy in children with autism, to providing aural rehabilitation and speech-language therapy for children with permanent hearing loss. She also has the unenviable pleasure of being speech-language pathologist for one of my children, whom Suzanne identified as having rather significant language delay. In my family, through our journey as parents of a child with speech-language delay, Suzanne raised a red flag that our daughter's ongoing constipation was not "just what many children go through," as our well-intended pediatrician told us. At Suzanne's gentle but strong recommendation, we sought further medical evaluations and discovered our daughter has celiac disease (an immune disorder characterized by a gluten intolerance, resulting in intestinal inflammation and inability to absorb nutrients from food). At the time of this writing, my family is finding the new normal that includes a gluten-free diet for one of our children. If not for Suzanne's incredible clinical intuition, our daughter would continue to struggle with constipation, the pain from which almost certainly has been a factor in her speech-language delays.

In an ideal world, a whole-family approach to addressing childhood speech-language disorders includes a highly insightful clinician, parents/caregivers who are engaged advocates, and a motivated child. Each participant (the speech-language pathologist, parent, and child) is influenced by the others. This book serves to provide parents with the tools necessary to engage with their child's clinicians to improve the likelihood that this team approach to speech and language intervention is optimized.

Brian J. Fligor, ScD, PASC

# ACKNOWLEDGMENTS

Writing this book has allowed me to fulfill a dream that I have had since the beginning of my career back in 1994. When I began this project eighteen months ago, I had only a shade of understanding about what I was about to do, and how it would change me. As I reflect now on the completion of this process, I am filled with gratitude for the many people who have helped me along the way.

First, I would like to thank Brian Fligor, my friend, my colleague, and my editor. I am so grateful that from the crowd of speech language pathologists that he knows, he chose me to work with on this book series. I can only hope that I have lived up to your expectations and to the example set by your book. Thank you for your help and support, your patience and your feedback. I know that it made my book better.

Further, I am grateful to Suzanne Staszak-Silva of Rowman & Littlefield for the opportunity to write a book, and for her patience and support throughout this process. And special thanks to Melissa McNitt for guiding me through the editing process with humor; I sincerely have enjoyed working with you.

Next, I would like to thank Mary Ellen Curran, a dear friend and colleague, for her thoughtful and helpful feedback. Mary Ellen is the clinician's clinician, and she sets the highest example for family-centered practice. I have no doubt that you pushed me to a higher standard. And to Danielle Mastrangelo, my niece and protégée, who provided a younger clinician's perspective. Thanks, D, for helping your Auntie out.

Taking on a project like this requires sacrifices from those closest to me as well. I want to thank Jeff MacFarlane, my partner and best friend, for supporting me and allowing me to take all the time I needed to get this done. Thank you for holding up both ends of the sky at times, and for being patient with all of the challenges that have come up, especially at the end of this year. I love you and I could not have done this without you.

From a longer-term perspective, I would like to thank my parents, Donald and Anna Ducharme. Mom and Dad, thank you for your unwavering faith, for supporting me while I pursued my education, and for your encouragement throughout my career. *This book is dedicated in part to you, for all that you are and for all that you have given me.*

Finally, I would like to offer my heartfelt gratitude and love to all of the children and families I have worked with in the past twenty-two years. You have taught me so much about the nature of love, family, and resilience, and you have pushed me and challenged me and trusted me to walk with you through some of the most difficult moments in your lives. My love for all of you knows no bounds. *This book is also dedicated to all of you, with the hope that I have given you just a fraction of what you have shared with me.*

# Part I

# I

# WELCOME TO THE JOURNEY

"**W**elcome to Holland" is a well-known story written by Emily Perl Kingsley,[1] a parent of a child with special needs. It speaks so well to the shock, the pain, and the betrayal of discovering that there is something wrong with your child. As you face the reality of a shift in your expectations and your dreams, and begin to tackle the logistical aspects of what comes next, you realize you are in a place you never dreamed you would be. There are so many questions about how and why this has happened, what it means for the future, and how you will make sense of this for yourself and everyone around you. You may have come to this place through many different doors:

- You always knew something was off. Perhaps even during pregnancy, you felt it was different, or you had dreams that made you uneasy;
- You have another child with developmental issues and hoped that it would not—could not—happen twice;
- You or your spouse have been in denial, not wanting to see the signs;
- You have found yourself endlessly comparing your child to others, or looking up developmental information on the Internet, with a growing sense of fear.

However, you have arrived; welcome to Where You Are. It may seem that you won't be able to handle it, or you may wonder how you will, but you know that there is a child here, one who needs your love and support and all the resources you have to offer. This book is for you. And for your family members, therapists, and friends who want to understand this journey you are on, this book will provide helpful information and guidance.

I stand with you. I am here to provide information, support, ideas, and resources. I am here to witness and to validate your own journey as a parent of a child with special needs. You have to be willing to "go there" with your own stuff, in order to move forward with your child and to learn to tell a new story. In my experience, the parents who invest as much in their own self-care and in processing their own complicated feelings and needs do much better in the long term. They are able to cultivate the resources they need; they are stronger advocates and tend to be healthier and better role models for their families. While the journey is not an easy one, and rarely follows a straight path, there can be healing and joy along the way.

## WHAT IS COMMUNICATION?

Communication—the ability to express oneself and to be understood—is one of life's most fundamental joys. It is often taken for granted until it is compromised through illness or injury. This is especially true for children, as it is usually assumed that language will emerge on its own with little effort. Yet, for millions of children each year, developing the skills that encompass communication, including speech and language skills, as well as attention and listening, stall or fail to develop at all. Even a mild disorder or temporary interruption in development can have long-term effects. These challenges can cause a wide variety of serious and far-reaching deficits that touch every aspect of a child's life. It is estimated that 7 percent of all children have Specific Language Impairment (a deficit in speech and language skills that is not explained by an underlying diagnosis or learning disability.[2] In addition, the rates of prematurity and autism spectrum disorders (ASD) continue to rise, causing many more children to have difficulty with the development of their communication skills.[3] As many as 10 percent of all children born annually will experience lifelong challenges related to a communication disorder.[4] It is the miraculous ability to communicate that we will learn about in this book.

## MY STORY

I have been blessed to work with some amazing families in over twenty years as a pediatric speech language pathologist (SLP). I have received as much as I have given from my "kids" and their families. I have been exposed to cultures and traditions from all over the globe, including those of India, Africa, Russia, Ecuador, China, Vietnam, Japan, France, and many more. Each family has shown me a slightly different version of the Journey, but all these families had threads in common. Regardless of the diagnosis, or the severity, it seems that families progress through a common path of questions and emotions, fears and triumphs. I am writing this book to share all that I have learned with you, to give you guidance, and to let you know that many have walked the path before you. You are not alone.

I am the youngest of six children, born to parents who highly valued education and reading. From a young age, I was a voracious reader, allowing me to build an enviable vocabulary. Beyond just learning words, communication was valued in my family. My parents modeled how to negotiate conflicts; my siblings were always close and had many friends. Talking at the dinner table was an epic affair, even when it was only a Tuesday night. It is a running joke in my family that people would line up to come to dinner at my house because you never knew who might be there or what topics might be covered. As a child, I loved the spoken word. I would spend hours, alone or with friends, talking, playing school, and building imaginary cities in the forts we built in the woods.

In elementary school, I had my first opportunity to be on stage. I played a wisecracking pumpkin in a play written by my third-grade class. I was hooked. What was better than the opportunity to communicate, to express myself, than to be on stage with a captive audience? Theater and music played an important role in my high school experience, challenging and stretching me to use my skills in new ways. I guess you could say I took it for granted that this ability was everyone's equal potential. I never conceived of not being able to speak or to connect with others in this way.

When I thought about my future, and what I would be, all of my vocational dreams centered around occupations that used communication as a core—lawyer, teacher, and writer. I was not sure what to pursue in college because none of those careers resonated with me on a deeper level. All of that changed my freshman year of college. I was at the University of Hartford, feeling like a fish out of water. I took the standard classes one takes in college, where you are allowed to cast about, looking for that topic or course that gets you. My *AHA* moment came in an exploratory class called "Freshman Dialogue."

Let's be honest. This was the university's way of checking up on its first-year students, who can be lost in so many ways during those first months away from home. For me, this class was a life changer. Mr. Smith was a guidance counselor at heart. He loved to give personality tests, aptitude tests, and any other kind of measure that would print out in a neat box who we were and what we were supposed to do. Every test he gave me, including the Meyers-Briggs Personality Type test,[5] listed speech language pathology as an ideal career for my skills and talents. Traits such a deep desire to serve others, compassion and warmth, and a quiet and serious nature made me a good candidate for speech language pathology.[6] My organizational skills, attention to detail, and an ability to observe a person or situation and design a plan to fill the gaps or needs would also be utilized in a very positive and important way as an SLP. [7]

Even though I had never heard of speech language pathology, there was a feeling, a resonance that I had never felt before. Today I know it as my intuitive abilities, guiding me in my life; it is an integral part of who I am as a clinician. As I began to explore just what this profession was, and to feel myself moving in that direction, that sense of purpose became clear for me. The following fall, after transferring to a school with a major in communication disorders, those initial feelings were confirmed. On the first day of my "Introduction to Communication Disorders" class at the University of Massachusetts Amherst, my professor, Dr. Ruth Huntley, began speaking about this profession and her clinical work as an SLP, everything came together. She described SLP as the intersection of art and science, something that I have embraced over and over during my career. This job requires nothing less than the most artful delivery of skills and techniques. It involves understanding cutting-edge science and traditional frameworks, and it involves being of service to others at a most vulnerable time in their lives.

I had always thought that I would work with adults. I was never good with kids, not even when I was one. Throughout my graduate training, I always envisioned myself working with adults, helping those who had lost their ability to communicate to regain it. I even accepted a job with a rehabilitation company a few weeks before my graduation from Emerson College, where I completed my master's degree. Fate intervened again, however, starting with a phone call from the Braintree Hospital Pediatric Center in Braintree, Massachusetts. That intuitive feeling prompted me to go and interview there, even though I had already secured a job. Within minutes, I knew that my plans were about to change. A few weeks later, I began my residency, called a Clinical Fellowship Year, and began working in a place where I would be immersed in clinical experiences, surrounded by many seasoned therapists who would guide the early development of my professional life.

I had the most interesting caseload, children who had all kinds of *diagnoses*; I was assigned to work with children who had had premature or difficult births, children who were late talkers, and many with a variety of other kinds of speech and language disorders. I was able to learn so much from these children and their families. Further, those experiences led me to develop many of the specialties that I now have and made me the clinician that I am today.

From the Pediatric Center, I moved to the neonatal intensive care unit (NICU) at a local hospital. This was a whole new experience for me. Given the expertise I had in feeding, swallowing, and early communication, working in the NICU was a natural next step. Although there are many challenges in working in this environment as an SLP, I deepened my understanding of *embryology* (the study of how babies develop in utero), *neurology* (the study of the brain), and many of the medical aspects of my field. At the same time, I was in the early stages of developing a private practice. At that time, I did all home-based care, primarily for an early intervention program in my area. This allowed me to work with many children, who were born prematurely, and to take my knowledge in related areas and bring them together.

Currently, I am the proud owner of South Shore Speech Pathology Partners, a busy private practice in Weymouth, Massachusetts. My practice caters to children with a variety of complex medical and developmental challenges. I also work with children who have difficulty in getting their communication skills going, who used to be called "late talkers." I have found a special affinity for working with these children and their families because they so often thrive and catch up to their peers. I am able to facilitate their "second birth," their emergence from a world of silence and frustration, to being an active participant in their family and community.

And my practice continues to grow and expand. In 2008, I began another journey that has fundamentally shifted the way that I practice as an SLP. I began taking classes in craniosacral therapy, or CST, a light-touch treatment typically thought to be the purview of physical and occupational therapists. Ironically, I began taking these classes out of a sense of obligation. I saw so many children who had a variety of different medical problems, such as reflux, food allergies, and constipation. So many times, parents would tell me that the doctors told them it was just "part of the diagnosis" and "something they would have to deal with." How could anyone "deal with" chronic pain or discomfort and also be expected to learn and master many new skills? Especially when they lacked the ability to tell people when they have just had enough? I wanted to be able to provide something more—something that could help these children *feel* better, not just get better at speech and language tasks.

CST has provided that tool. It is based on the premise that it is possible to normalize and soothe the nervous system and to clear restrictions that inhibit normal growth, development, and learning.[8] The children whom I shared CST with seemed to attend better, to retain better; I also often hear parents say that they seem calmer, and sometimes even sleep better. In my intensive study of both CST and SLP, I have learned that "stressed systems don't strengthen."[9] This means that when we are trying to learn a new skill, establish a new habit, or do any task that pushes our nervous system past its current state, we must be in a "just right" place to make that leap. If we are ill, exhausted, dehydrated, emotionally distressed, or in any way compromised, it becomes impossible for our brains to do that work. We simply are not made that way. However, we routinely demand of children with developmental challenges that they push themselves to the limit and beyond. Our interventions, which are necessary and well intentioned, can also be a source of further stress to an already damaged system. CST provides the antidote and a way to provide positive, supportive touch, which we all crave. It gives the body and the brain a chance to reset and to function more normally. Learning overlaid on a better functioning system is going to happen with less effort, and yield better and longer lasting results.

CST has also allowed me to work on a deeper level because it has changed me as a person. What I have found is that CST can be a catalyst for children because it allows them to be more neurologically available for the traditional SLP work that I offer. It allows them to process experiences and to build neural frameworks that underlie both successful communication and learning. Is it a silver bullet? No, nothing is. But what it does do is open the possibility for children to learn more or differently than they would have without it. And that can make all the difference.

CST is considered an "alternative therapy," developed by Dr. John Upledger, an osteopath, in the 1960s. He discovered that there is a rhythmic movement in the fluids and membranes surrounding the brain and spinal cord, or what CST practitioners would call the craniosacral system. Dr. Upledger expanded on the work of others who had investigated and studied the bones in the head and how they move and are impacted by compression and compromise. He then developed an entire framework and approach that allowed trained practitioners to locate and treat issues in the body using a series of holds and release techniques that allow the body to realign and heal itself. As practitioners, we tune into the Inner Wisdom or Inner Physician in each of our clients and activate and facilitate his or her own natural healing abilities. One of the reasons that I was drawn to CST is that I am not forcing anything. I am working with the client's own body and helping to create an opportunity to help his or her own nervous system. [10]

Dr. Upledger spent many years working with biomedical engineers, therapists, and others to conduct research into the impact and efficacy of this new therapy and to document via objective means what he could feel happening in the body. Research continues actively today, to determine how CST can help those with concussion, [11] autism, [12] and other conditions. Like any protocol or technique that is designed to be used with sick or otherwise vulnerable people, CST has had its critics and those who may not be aware of its basis in anatomy and physiology, and science and medicine. There are even some who call it a fraud. This is common in the development of new therapies and scientific discoveries; you would be hard pressed to find anything now commonly accepted in scientific circles that was not rigorously challenged, especially if that discovery meant shifting what had been considered absolute truths.

So, CST continues to undergo questioning and will continue to develop its research base. This is welcome and necessary. However, even as an SLP, I can tell you that basic research is often five to ten years behind clinical practice. And even the tenets of evidenced-based practice, a requirement that services be provided to clients based on tiers of hard scientific evidence, includes a space for clinician experience and client results and judgments.[13] In my practice, I offer CST when I feel it is clinically indicated and relevant. I discuss the potential benefits and risks with the client or parents, and they make the choice to try or to continue with CST as part of the treatment plan. The parents participate in setting goals, and we monitor to see if those goals are being met. We work together to determine whether CST has a valid place in the treatment program and whether they feel it helps them, as parents, or the child *feel and function* better.

In the past several years, I have noticed that my work has shifted yet again. I have come to the awareness that I am working as much, if not more in some cases or moments in time, with parents and families. This is most typically the mother, but can be any significant caregiver in a child's life. I have even had parents who bravely ventured into dealing with their own emotions and issues after seeing the difference that CST made for their child. These women wanted to process their own feelings and develop better coping skills so that they could be there for their child in a deeper way. And they are inspirational. My practice now reflects the gradual shift that I have made from working with the child alone to working with the family around that child. This might include parents, grandparents, siblings, and others. I work to honor and support the context in which the child exists every day, as well as the layers of relationship and interaction that impact how that child is able to function and see him- or herself as they grow and develop.

## WHY I AM WRITING THIS BOOK

I am writing this book as a love letter to all the children and families that I have worked with in the past twenty-two years. I am writing this book as an invitation to those who find themselves beginning the journey now. I believe in the healing power of honesty, clarity, validation, and support. I hope to create a space where you can learn about your child's issues, but also honor your own. I want to provide you with information and, hopefully, answer some of your questions about speech and language development and disorders. Beyond that, I want to connect you virtually with the millions of other parents who have stood in your place, and to those who will come after you. This book serves as a resource and guide for you to develop some of the skills and traits that you may need to be a successful, even joyful parent.

When you feel validated and supported, you can face your emotions, honor them, process them, and Get On With It. Given the correct information and resources, you can be a more aware parent, advocate, and model. And perhaps most importantly, when you take the time to invest in your emotional health and well-being, your physical health is better. As any parent knows, your health and well-being are directly related to your ability to manage stress, cope with short- and long-term challenges, and handle the logistics of a busy and often complex life.

Having a child with special needs provides additional stresses that go beyond those experienced by parents of typically developing children. Many parents report they experience increased anxiety, depression, marital stress, more frequent illnesses, sleep disturbances, and other stress-related challenges. If stress is not managed well, it can eventually result in more serious illnesses, such as heart disease and obesity, and it can increase the occurrence of digestive issues (reflux and ulcers) and other conditions such as migraines and chronic pain.[14] These facts make it clear that taking care of yourself physically and emotionally has broad implications for you and for your family. So I offer you this invitation.

## HOW TO USE THIS BOOK

Take the time to read this book. Use part I to learn about speech and language development, the role of speech language pathologists, common disorders, and types of intervention for speech and language challenges. This is the part of the book with information you can use and share with others. Part II is just for you. Think of it as your own project in development. You can use the guided experiences and questions to go deeper into the emotional side; challenge yourself to validate your own feelings and to reach for healing. You could also use this section of the book as part of a support group, working with other parents in similar situations, or as part of your work with a therapist or social worker who can provide further support as you move along. While this book is not intended to diagnose or treat any particular issue, or to replace the need for a skilled therapist, it can provide you with basic information and support to get you started. It can also help you determine where more help is needed.

It is my sincere hope that you will find this book helpful and useful. I encourage you to reach out to spouses, family members, friends, and others who can support you in your desire to become a *thriving* parent of a child with special needs.

# 2

# ALPHABET SOUP AND SEEING YOUR CHILD IN CONTEXT

Learning to "speak the language" is a key factor in the success of any new endeavor, whether it is a new hobby, a foreign travel adventure, or starting a new job or profession. Walking within the world of special education and medical issues is no different. Understanding the terminology and being able to keep up with the professionals who are working with your child allows you to successfully navigate meetings and evaluations, and provides you with the confidence that you need to make decisions and guide the process. In short, it empowers you as the leader of the team working with your child, and it demonstrates your mastery. Yet, many times, I have seen parents struggle to make sense of an endless stream of acronyms and professional terminology, becoming more and more stressed and overwhelmed as a meeting or report progresses. This is combined with the already taxing task of processing the *underlying content* of what is being said about your child and what it means about his or her future.

This chapter is designed to provide you with a basic primer of terms used in speech language pathology, as well as some common terms in the medical arena and special education. You may want to begin keeping a book of terms related to your child's diagnosis or treatment, and add to it as needed. In addition, you should speak up when terms are used that you don't understand. It is your right to have all the information and to be able to put it in context so that you understand how it relates to the bigger picture of your child's development or function.

First, let's talk about the most fundamental terms in speech language pathology, and how they are often confused and substituted for one another.

**What Is Speech?** In simple terms, speech is movement made audible. It is the act of producing speech sounds using the mouth, sometimes called *articulation* or *speech production*. Speech is produced through the coordinated use of four systems in the body: *respiration*, *phonation* (or *"voicing"*), *resonance*, and *articulation*. When we prepare to speak, we inhale (take air in) and close our vocal cords. The air coming up from our lungs (**respiration**) meets the resistance of the closed vocal cords, and the pressure that builds up causes the vocal cords to begin vibrating (**voicing**). The speed and tension that is present when the vibration occurs dictates the pitch and quality of the voice; loudness is determined by the amount of pressure generated from the air stream. As the sound of the vibration travels up to the nose and mouth, it takes on the qualities of various sounds depending on the shape of the vocal tract (**resonance)** and where the sound is allowed to flow (such as open sounds or vowels) or is stopped, as in most consonant sounds (**articulation.)**

In order to understand this, close your eyes and prepare to say "Hi." Notice that you take a breath in and begin to exhale. The whole vocal tract is open for the /h/ sound, and then you turn your voice on for the vowel /ai/ (a long i sound.) Notice that when you produce the /h/, your mouth is already pulling your lips back for the /ee/ (long e) sound at the end of the word *Hi*. Now observe what happens when you say "hot." While your mouth may start in the same position as for *Hi*, your mouth changes shape for the /o/ (short o sound in hot) vowel, and then you stop the air with your tongue behind your front teeth for the /t/. Try this with "map". . . your nose is open to allow for production of the /m/, while your mouth changes shape again for the "a" vowel sound in the middle, while you stop the air at your lips for the /p/. It is truly a marvel how complex speech production is when you think about it!

These skills can be directly assessed, and their development follows a typical path, with sounds emerging at different ages (see appendix A). Speech is often described with words such as "clarity" or "intelligibility," and when there is a speech sound disorder, it is usually given a severity level from mild to severe. According to the National Outcomes

Measurement System from the American Speech-Language-Hearing Association (ASHA), a mild articulation disorder is described as "consistently understood by familiar people and usually understood by unfamiliar listeners. The child's speech calls attention to itself more than would be expected for the child's age and it occasionally affects participation in adult-child, peer and directed group activities." In contrast, a severe articulation disorder is described as "speech that cannot be understood even by familiar listeners."[1]

As an example, John is a four-year-old boy who has a frontal lisp, meaning he uses the sound /th/ for /s/. Although this might be visually distracting, his speech can still be understood by most people, even if they do not know him well. In contrast, Jane is a three-year-old girl who can only produce the sounds /b/ and /uh/, and she uses this syllable to mean everything. Her speech would not be understood easily even by those who know her best, requiring a lot of context cues and practice by her communication partners.

**What Is Language?** Many people think about speech and language as being one and the same, but they are in fact very different. While speech is a *motor* activity, language is a *cognitive* one. Language includes the ideas that we express, and the words and sentences we use to express them. It can be verbal when words are used, but it can also be nonverbal, including gestures, facial expressions, and sign language, or it can be written. Most of the time, we use a combination of verbal and nonverbal means to express ourselves, such as how we use our tone of voice or facial expression to convey the mood behind our words, or how we can say the same exact sentence but mean something entirely different when we want to convey sarcasm or a question.

We typically look at two aspects of language that provide us with useful information. The first is *receptive language*, which is our understanding and comprehension of language. This includes skills such as vocabulary; concept development; and being able to process and understand directions, recall information, and follow stories and conversation. It refers to how we are able to attach meaning to the words we hear, and comprehend what we hear in order to learn and produce responses. In our first few years, we learn thousands of single words, and some of these words relate to various aspects of other words, or how words relate to one another. An example of this is concepts. Children must master many types of concepts in order to successfully process and understand language. This is true for following directions in the home and, especially, later when learning in school. Examples of these include spatial concepts (*in, on, under, behind, next to*—words that describe location and spatial relationships between things), descriptive concepts (*wet, red, sticky, big, scary*—words that describe the physical and sensory aspects of objects) and quantitative concepts (*more, less*, and numbers—words that describe numerical relationships and allow comparison).

In contrast, *expressive language* refers to the output side of language. Expressive language can most easily be thought of as having three primary parts:[2]

**Content:** *Content* is the *substance* of what we express. It includes the words and vocabulary, but mainly it is about our ideas and the meaning we are trying to convey. When we think about children, we ask questions such as:

- What is he or she trying to tell me?
- How meaningful are the attempts to communicate?
- How easy is it to understand the message? How clear is their meaning?

**Form:** *Form* refers to the way that we *package our deeper message.* This includes things like grammar, word order, and word retrieval (being able to come up with the specific word you want). It is possible to convey a message clearly, even if the form is off. This is typical for toddlers and older children with language challenges, who often miss words, or get the grammar wrong, but you still know what they want. Many children struggle with the form of their communication, even though they know what they want to say. When we think about form, we ask questions such as:

- Has the child mastered the structure of language/grammar as expected for their age?
- Is he able to easily and effectively communicate his message?
- How do his articulation skills impact this area?

Many times, children who have articulation issues will be slow to master the *form* of communication until they are able to produce the later-developing sounds that are so common in our expression of grammar. For example, children who have difficulty with the production of sounds such as /s/ (a sound not often mastered until 3.5 or 4 years of age) do not mark plural and possessives with accuracy; it is up to the SLP to determine whether the error is solely related to an articulation delay or a linguistic delay.

**Use:** *Use* refers to *how* and *why* children use their verbal and non-verbal language skills. It considers the human context in which language is used and is sometimes referred to as "social communication." When looking at this area, SLPs must ask themselves questions such as:

- Why does this child communicate? We look for three general purposes: to regulate the behavior of another person (requesting, calling, protesting), to establish joint attention (greeting, labeling, commenting), or to have social interaction (playing social games, sharing ideas).
- How easily does she engage with others?
- How readily does she engage with others?
- How frequently does she attempt to interact with others (rate of communication)? This considers how frequently a child *initiates* communication with others, and it is a measure of intention level and how confident she is in establishing communication with others. Children who exhibit a low rate of communication are often more of a concern than those children who frequently *try*, regardless of how successful they are.

In looking at *content, form and use*, we are able to obtain a fairly comprehensive picture of a child's linguistic competence. When we combine this with their clarity of speech, their understanding, and their cognitive skills and attention, we begin to understand each child's total communication competence.

**What Is Communication?** *Communication* is the umbrella term that includes all the areas outlined above; it refers to children's ability to navigate their world and to use their *speech and language* abilities to influence and impact others. It is a complex and multilayered profile that provides a window into how well children are able to manage their daily lives. In young children, this refers most specifically to how children learn to use words to get what they want, and how they learn to understand their world. For older children, they learn to use their language to build social relationships and to master academic curriculum. Each has its own purpose and its own challenges.

**Other useful terminology related to speech language pathology:**

**Voice:** How well we make voice, including pitch, loudness, and quality. Common difficulties in this area include vocal nodules, chronic hoarseness, and laryngitis. This refers to the structures of the throat and voice box and how well it works.

**Fluency:** This refers to how easily we are able to produce speech. Dysfluency, commonly referred to as *stuttering*, refers to difficulties in coordinating airflow and speaking so that there are frequent interruptions in the flow of speech. These may show up as sound or word repetitions, prolonged sounds, and difficulty initiating speech at all. There are many theories about the causes and best treatments for stuttering, which are beyond the scope of this book. See the references section at the back of the book.

**Articulation:** As noted above, *articulation* refers specifically to the production of speech sounds and whether or not the child is using them as expected, given the child's age, neurological, and oral motor status.

**Oral Motor Skills:** Relates to the structures and functions of the mouth used for speaking and feeding. This includes the jaw, the tongue, lips, teeth, and palate. We consider muscle tone, motor ability, and the quality of movements.

**Speech Language Pathologist:** A professional with an advanced degree, (at least a master's degree) in speech pathology. SLPs are licensed in most states, and most possess the Certificate of Clinical Competence (CCC) from the American Speech-Language-Hearing Association (ASHA.)

**Speech Language Pathology Assistant (SLPA):** A trained paraprofessional who operates under the direct supervision of a certified SLP, to assist in the provision of services to client/patients/students. Assistants typically have a bachelor's degree in communication disorders or a related field and have training in specific and defined aspects of clinical service provision. They are not nationally credentialed at this time but may be licensed by the state in which they practice. Assistants may not represent themselves as SLPs, nor do the work of an SLP.

**Physical Therapist (PT):** A professional who typically holds an advanced degree (master's degree or higher) and is licensed by the state and nationally certified. Physical therapists generally work on balance, coordination, and gross motor skills for safety and mobility.

**Physical Therapy Assistant (PTA):** A trained paraprofessional who works under the direction and supervision of a licensed PT. PTAs are required to earn an associate's degree and are also licensed and certified.

**Occupational Therapist (OT):** A professional who has earned an advanced degree (master's degree) and also has state licensure and national certification. OTs work on functional skills for daily living, although the OT profession often overlaps with other professions to work on areas such as feeding. OTs also address sensory integration issues, productivity, and hand function.

**Occupational Therapy Assistant (OTA):** A health care paraprofessional who works under the direction of an OT to carry out specific exercises or treatment plans. OTAs are required to have an associate's degree and be certified.

**Sensory Processing Disorder/Sensory Integration (SPD/SI):** This refers to our brain's ability to take in information from all the senses and produce adaptive responses that allow us to interact functionally with our environment. When there is a problem with the ability to manage sensory input from one or more systems, SPD or SI dysfunction may be diagnosed.

**Audiologist:** A licensed and frequently board-certified professional who has obtained an advanced degree in audiology. They perform hearing testing and provide diagnostic services and sometimes hearing-aid fitting for children and adults. In some states, educational audiologists provide direct consultation to school districts to support children with hearing loss in the classroom.

**Autism Spectrum Disorders (ASD):** The umbrella term for disorders of social communication and cognition; also called "pervasive developmental disorders" (PDD).

**Augmentative and Alternative Communication (AAC):** The collection of technologies and strategies used to support or replace verbal communication for those who cannot speak.

**Applied Behavioral Analysis (ABA):** A structured approach used in the education of children with autism spectrum disorders and others with specific needs; ABA uses discrete trial training and reinforcement to assist children with building the skills needed for learning.

**American Sign Language (ASL):** A language used by members of the deaf community; ASL has its own word order, grammatical structure, and culture.

**Specific Language Impairment (SLI):** The presence of a language disorder when there is no hearing loss or other developmental delays.

**Traumatic Brain Injury (TBI):** Any injury to the skull or brain that can result in mild to severe cognitive deficits.

**Individual Family Service Plan (IFSP):** The contract made between families of children in early intervention and the service providers. It typically includes history, evaluation results, and a service-delivery plan.

**Early Intervention (EI):** A federally mandated program for children from birth to three years of age with developmental needs. A variety of developmental services may be provided, within the context of a family-driven model.

**Individual Education Plan (IEP):** The contract document that outlines service delivery for children served in the public school system, between three and twenty-one years of age. It typically includes history, vision statement, evaluation information, accommodations, and strategies and service delivery information. It is reviewed on an annual basis or as needed.

**Attention Deficit Disorder/Attention Deficit Hyperactivity Disorder (ADD/ADHD):** A cluster of disorders initially seen in childhood that causes difficulty with attention and focus. There are several subtypes, depending on the primary symptoms seen.

**(Central) Auditory Processing Disorder ([C]APD):** A cluster of disorders that result from a breakdown somewhere between the auditory neural pathways and the auditory cortex in the brain, usually in the presence of normal hearing. It defines how well spoken language is transferred from the ear to the brain and understood. (C)APD relates to difficulty with processing and managing speech sounds and understanding in the presence of background noise. It is diagnosed by an audiologist and may be treated by an SLP. It usually requires a combination of environmental modifications and direct treatment.

**Learning Disabilities (LD):** A cluster of disorders that relate to the ability to understand and manage information, usually in the presence of average or above average intelligence.

**Childhood Apraxia of Speech (CAS):** Also known as *dyspraxia*. A significant speech disorder that results from difficulty in programming the sounds for speech. Children with CAS often have normal intelligence and good receptive language skills but have difficulty getting information from the motor area of the brain to the mouth intact. CAS is also a spectrum, with symptoms ranging from mild to severe.

**Within Normal Limits (WNL):** Indicates that a child's test scores or functioning are within expected ranges for age/grade level.

**Within Functional Limits (WFL):** Indicates that a child's test scores or skills are functional for their age/grade, or approaching normal ranges.

**TX/RX:** A common medical abbreviation for *treatment* or *rehabilitation*.

**HX:** A common medical abbreviation for *history*.

**DX:** A common medical abbreviation for *diagnosis*.

**NOS:** A common medical abbreviation for *not otherwise specified*. Indicates that a child may not meet all the criteria for a particular diagnosis, or that normal results were found.

**Failure to Thrive (FTT):** Indicates that a child's weight or rate of growth is below expectations for their age. Usually weight is less than the third percentile for children at a given age.

**CP:** Medical abbreviation for *cerebral palsy*, a cluster of disorders resulting from brain injury around the time of birth; it may affect one or both sides of the body and cause high or low muscle tone.

**CA:** Abbreviation for *chronological age*. It may also be followed by corrected age in the case of a child born prematurely.

**DOS:** Abbreviation for *date of service* or *date of summary*; used in reports.

**GDD:** Abbreviation for global developmental delay. This refers to significant delays and deficits that affect a child across multiple systems: cognitive, motor, and communication.

**Standard Deviation (SD):** Refers to how a child's scores on a formal, standardized test relate to the performance of same age peers on the same test.

**Hypo:** A prefix noting something below the threshold of what would be expected, as in hypotonia (low muscle tone) or hypoarousal (low state of alertness).

**Hyper:** A prefix indicating something above the threshold of what would be expected, as in hypertonia (high or spastic muscle tone) or hyperarousal (high state of alertness).

## SEEING THE CHILD IN CONTEXT

We exist in our lives by playing a number of roles over time. Some are fixed, such as woman/man or youngest child, while others change over time, such as spouse, parent, coach, or your professional title. Understanding the roles of family members and appreciating the layers of relationships, agendas, and needs can bring clarity and guide decision making. In looking at children with developmental challenges, I find it helpful to think about three distinct contexts through which we can view their roles, strengths, and challenges: the *biological* context, the *social* context, and the *therapeutic* context.

The first context is the biological context. This includes information relative to genetics, the complete medical history and profile, and the trajectory of development. Let's look at each one in turn. Genetics is a prime topic for research and innovation at this moment in time. While we have always been taught to believe that our genes are fixed and represent the core of the hand nature has dealt, we now know that there is hope for gene therapy or other medical advances that could not have been imagined even ten years ago. Exciting research is now examining the connection between genes and the environment, as it relates to the expression of our genes. For our purposes, it is important to know if there is a genetic component to a child's presentation. Is there a syndrome or diagnosis that has a clearly identified risk for speech and language issues? Or is there a strong family connection to the particular issue, such as many male cousins who stutter, or several children in the family who had language delays or feeding issues? This will help provide some information about what outcomes we may be able to expect, as well as what may have been helpful in terms of intervention.

Within the biological context, we also want to look at the complete medical picture as well. While the genes are the canvas, the medical history and presentation provide the paint. We want to consider all aspects of medical experience, including illnesses, allergies, surgeries, or medical interventions and diagnoses. It is possible that the treatment for a primary diagnosis can cause a secondary problem; one example of this is seen in children with seizure disorders. The medications given to stop or control seizures can often result in feeding and swallowing issues, as these medications are meant to suppress the nervous system, including the muscles needed to safely swallow. We also want to consider the health and functioning of all the organ systems in the body, as well as the immune system. Many children who have challenges in development also have increased rates of illness and battle colds and infections frequently. Frequent ear infections can cause hearing loss and increase the risk of speech and language delays. Severe reflux and food allergies can cause delays in feeding skills, poor nutrition, and aversion. Long-term implications include possible vocal cord pathology and cognitive delays.

Finally, we want to look at the developmental picture as part of the biological context. While genetics and the medical profile are critical elements of this, we must also consider the total picture of development for the child. This includes both where he is *now* and how his development has progressed from the time of conception. We want to think about the global picture of his development, as well as all of the individual contributing factors. For example, perhaps you have a child who has no significant medical history, but he is presenting with significant speech and language issues. Or, in contrast, you have a daughter who was born prematurely after a difficult pregnancy and delivery and who has been plagued by allergies, feeding issues, ear infections, and reflux. How we approach diagnosis and treatment for the resulting speech and language disorder would need to take into account all the other pieces of the puzzle in order to have the best results.

The second context that we consider is the *social* context. This is how we view the child in light of their relationships and settings. First, we want to consider the family. Every child exists within a family unit, which may include one or two parents, siblings, aunts, uncles, cousins, grandparents . . . and each one of them has a view of the family as a whole and each member within it. The family as a whole has defined (although perhaps unwritten) roles and strategies that it uses to function. Having a child with a disability, or even a developmental delay, can cause upset within the system and lead to difficulties in communication and interaction. I often hear from parents about the "helpful advice" they receive from well-meaning relatives and extended family about how their child will certainly catch up, or how easy it should be to just "handle" the situation. We want to consider the child within the whole family, including the quality of relationships and how supportive the extended family is to the nuclear family. We also want to consider how each family processes having a child with a disability, and how this impacts everyone's ability to accept and integrate a child into family functions and psychology.

Within the social context, we also want to consider the educational setting where a child receives her schooling. In addition to being the place where she spends most of her time, we want to consider therapies received, how and where she participates in educational activities, and how successfully she is participating in school, including the type and quality of her peer relationships. We want to consider your relationship as parent and advocate with the school and school personnel. How easily do you communicate your concerns to school staff? How well does school staff understand your child, in terms of both needs and special qualities?

Finally, we consider the greater community where your child resides as part of the social context. We look at neighborhoods, community activities, and resources. By understanding what is available in your community, we are able to establish goals for integrating your child into the larger context of family life.

The third context that we look at is the *therapeutic* context. This includes the community of educators and interventionists who work with your child. We look at their individual skills and experience, as well as their chemistry with your child. We want to consider your relationship to them as parent, too. As any therapist or parent who has participated in even five minutes of treatment can tell you, working with children involves chemistry and relationship as much as it does clinical skills. In addition to the individuals working with your child, we want to consider how well these professionals function as a team. Chances are, they may be spread out over different facilities and may have varied models for service delivery. It is important for you as the parent to be able to coordinate their services and their styles of interacting with your child. For treatment to be optimally successful, services should be integrated, and all team members should all be talking to one another regularly, via phone or e-mail, to stay on top of how things are progressing. Sometimes it is you, the parent, who must insist on this communication, and often you may have to coordinate it as well.

Although it may seem like a lot to consider, all of the factors described above are important in effectively diagnosing and treating children with a range of developmental challenges. A good therapist will ask questions and seek to understand the complete picture of your child in order to design a treatment plan that will help them participate in the totality of their life. By fully exploring your child's functioning within their biological, social, and therapeutic contexts, we come to appreciate the whole picture of who they are and are better able to help them move forward.

# 3

# COMMUNICATION DEVELOPMENT

This chapter will provide an in-depth review of the development of communication skills in children, including aspects of both speech and language. The chapter is divided into three sections: I. Brain and Overall Development, II. Stages of Speech and Language Development, and III. Supporting Speech and Language Development. I recommend using this chapter as a reference; you can refer to it to see how your child is progressing at a particular stage, or you can look to see what might be coming next.

Before we begin, I suggest that you take a moment to close your eyes and tune in to the miraculous nature of human communication. Just for a moment, think about the many ways that you communicate thoughts, feelings, and ideas throughout your day. You use gestures, facial expressions and body position, eye contact, words, and tone of voice as well as written language to communicate with others. When you pause to appreciate the complexity and the importance of communication, you begin to understand why children who have communication challenges are so globally impacted.

In fact, the ability to communicate, to understand the world, and to express oneself is one of the most important tasks that children undertake in the first five years of life. Children must master many foundational skills in order to become successful communicators. Difficulty in any one of these areas can have a significant impact on confidence and feelings of self-esteem. As a parent or caregiver, you are in a unique position to foster and enhance typical language development, as well as help to support your child who is struggling. This chapter will provide you with a solid understanding about the typical development of speech and language skills embedded in an understanding of how the brain develops. We will also discuss the relationship between sensory integration and communication skills. Later on, you'll be given examples of how you as a parent or family member can help your child to develop his or her communication skills.

Supporting children who are struggling with communication skills is not always obvious or intuitive, and becoming a good language facilitator takes thought and guidance. I hope to offer you some techniques that will work for your family. It is my hope that this chapter will assist you in becoming a wiser, savvier communication facilitator.

## I. BRAIN AND OVERALL DEVELOPMENT

### The Developing Brain

In order to understand how speech and language—and ultimately communication—develop, we can begin by thinking about the brain in a newborn baby. We are all born with more than 1 billion brain cells existing in various areas of the brain. Through the course of development, and especially in the first year, many of these brain cells will become associated and connected in vast and complex networks, while others will die off in a controlled process much like weeding a garden. This development is driven by experience: first by sensory experience and interacting with the world and then by cognitive process and learning.[1] Although we think of language as being centered in one area of the brain, the areas that are needed for successful communication, including speech and language, are actually found throughout the brain. At its core, helping a child develop speech language skills and become a confident communicator truly involves helping to shape their brain.

The brain is divided into two halves, the left and right; each half also has four *lobes,* or areas, with specialized functions. The **frontal lobe** sits behind our forehead and controls our emotions and our ability to plan and carry out tasks. You may have heard the term *executive function,* or *executive skills* in relation to this area. You can think of this lobe as the boss or CEO of your brain, controlling the way you approach tasks as well as overseeing production. When there is a problem in this area, children may have difficulty with emotional control and mood swings, as well as initiating and completing tasks.

The **temporal lobes** sit over the ears and house the parts of the brain that control hearing, understanding, and language processing. Problems in this area of the brain often result in problems with speech and language skills. Many adults who suffer a stroke have damage in this area, which causes the loss of communication ability.

The **parietal lobes** sit at the sides of the head, above the temporal lobes. The parietal lobes are responsible for our sensory experiences and the integration of information from all of our senses. Finally, the **occipital lobe** sits at the back of the head. Its main function relates to vision and the processing of visual information.

We also want to consider the *corpus collosum*, which is the band of fibers that connects the right and left sides of the brain. Information passes through this band of tissue constantly, helping the left and right sides work together. It is important to have a working corpus collosum so that we can integrate the best of both sides of the brain. Our left brain is most commonly associated with language and logical, linear thinking. It is the analytical part of our mind, the part that helps us with organization, details, and solving problems. It is the *doer*. In contrast, our right brain is more commonly associated with music, rhythm, color, and emotion. It is the part of us that focuses on the bigger picture, the whole picture, and the larger meaning of experiences. Right-brain function also includes intuition and qualities of *being*.

It is thought that we each have a *dominant* hemisphere that plays the role of leader and seems to dictate the way we respond to things. Bring to mind someone in your life who tends to approach everything as if it were a math equation or who falls back on logic even in times of stress. Contrast this with someone you know who sees the color of life and has an artistic and dreamy outlook. These are examples of what it means to be "left-brained," as in the first profile, and "right-brained," as in the second.[2] The truth is, we actually need both sides functioning well to fully participate in our lives and to navigate the full spectrum of our responsibilities. For children, this means having experiences that stimulate the development of both sides of the brain and having opportunities to learn to integrate skills across the body. There are a few other

aspects of brain development that are important to consider when looking at children:

- **Contralateral Control:** Each side of the body is controlled by
  the opposite side of the brain; difficulties in the left side of the
  brain will result in right-sided weakness or dysfunction.
- **Development of the Midline:** Children need to become aware
  of the center of their body in order to develop the skills that
  involve crossing over the midline. This includes skills such as
  reading (the eyes sweep from left to right), cutting, chewing (the
  tongue moves food from one side to the other), and many more.
- **Bilateral Control:** As part of developing a sense of the midline,
  and the ability to cross it functionally, children must learn to use
  two hands together. They must also learn to alternate hands and
  to do two different tasks simultaneously.

It is with this in mind that we will begin to talk about how skills
develop in young children.

## Stages of Typical Development

*General Principles*

It may be helpful to outline some general principles of language development before we look more specifically at the sequence. First, **there
is a wide range of normal or typical development**. For example,
first words can come anywhere between nine months and fourteen
months and still be considered within the normal range. As children are
developing so many skills in the first five years of life, where and when
they expend their brain resources on language or communication can
vary greatly. Further, **children move at their own pace through
each of the stages.** One of the most common things that I see with
children who are language impaired is that there may be big break-
throughs and skill development followed by a long period of integration, or what might be called "plateauing." This is where the child does
not seem to make a lot of progress for a period of time. I usually teach
parents to observe this as a *stair-step* approach to development. In fact
this may be your child's style of learning, one of many. The next princi-

ple is that **development is hierarchical and cumulative—you can't skip steps**. Just as children must crawl before they can successfully walk, children learning to communicate go through very predictable stages, with each one building on the one before, in a logical progression. It is important that a child experience each of the stages in order to reach her potential. And while many people know of a child who never crawled and yet still learned to walk, you may also be aware that she had other subtle deficits that followed from missing that stage of preparation in motor development.

Another particularly important principle is that **speech and language development and communication follow and result from the development of motor and play skills.** For many children, the development of the gross motor skills greatly impacts the speed and the quality of his or her ability to develop communication. This includes such things as the ability to hold the head and body upright so that it is possible to hold and play with toys, or the ability to move and rotate the trunk to allow better rib cage expansion for making sounds. Our expectations for what a child can do in some areas is directly impacted by how he is learning to use his body in space to move against gravity, for holding and manipulating objects. Next, **play is the work of children.** Language development directly follows from the type and quality of experiences a child has in play. Play allows a child to associate meaning with words and actions and forms the foundation on which she builds vocabulary, sentence structure, social interaction, and many other skills. Next, we must **consider the whole child and his or her overall development.** It is impossible to just look at how a child is learning to speak and understand when we must consider so many other aspects of her development as well. As noted above, the developing brain has limited cognitive resources during those first five years, and when the focus is intensified in one area (such as walking), the energy available for working on communication is minimized. Often, once a child masters walking, her communication skyrockets! The other important aspect of this principle is that we must look at the child as more than just the accumulation of words; we want to consider her development in total. This includes taking factors such as medical health, environment, and family stability and available resources into consideration.

Next, we want our **focus to be on communication and not just spoken words.** Many parents have a lot of anxiety about when a child will begin to speak words, how many words he has, or how successful he is in understanding language. A significant part of my work with very young children involves helping parents and children tune in to each other and realize the many ways that infants and young children communicate using a variety of nonverbal strategies. We must also look at the development of gestures and how a child attempts to use facial expressions and tone of voice to express himself. We also want to look at how frequently and why he communicates, that is, the rate and function of communication, because that gives us a sense of how he initiates communication and how he responds to an adult's efforts to communicate. Success depends on having *both in place and working well.*

Finally, we want to remember that **language is supposed to be fun and interactive**; it is a creative endeavor that allows for unique interactions with many people in various situations throughout the day. One of the most important parts of communication development is the gradual transition from just getting people to do what you want (behavioral regulation) to communicating and interacting for purely social purposes and they joy of shared experience. This is how a child comes to understand his power as a communicator.

### The Goals of Communication Development

Let's review some of the overall goals of communication development. First, a child must **develop all the prerequisite skills or foundation skills** that precede the development of speech and language. That child must also **develop attachment and secure relationships**, as this forms the basis for social interaction and provides the context for communication. Children **must also develop a vocabulary and a fund of knowledge** (an understanding of what things are and how they work) in order to have topics that are meaningful to communicate about. Children **must develop a sound system** and the ability to produce and combine sounds in ways that mirror and her native language. Children must also **learn how to express more complex ideas and thoughts** by learning to combine words and sentences using the rules of her native language. Children also need **learn the reasons why we communicate and be able to utilize all of them** successfully and easily. Finally, children must also **increase the rate of communica-**

**tion**, so that she is able to participate in a rapid exchange of information, such as in a conversation or social game.

## Foundation Skills Children Learn

What are the foundation skills that children must master in order to become successful communicators? First, children must develop what we call the "prerequisite" skills. These include things like joint attention, interaction, turn taking, imitation, and the motor skills that allow for spoken language. An explanation of each of these follows.

**Joint attention** is an expression of how readily the child is able to share an experience with a partner. It means one or more people looking at and experiencing something in the moment together. With infants, parents might tune in to a child by gazing into her eyes. An older child may initiate joint attention by inviting you to look at, label, or share something that he is interested in. As you might imagine, this skill is particularly important for the development of social communication because it involves a give and take, and a shared experience.

**Interaction** is what follows from joint attention. A child may ask what something is ("What is that?") or ask you to look at it ("See the plane, mama?"), or they may ask you to participate in some way in their discovery or experience of something ("Watch me go down the slide!"). This is directly related to the concept of **turn taking**, which happens even in the earliest moments after birth. Children learn to engage in cycles, using eye gaze, vocalization, and movement. The easy back-and-forth of cooing with your baby and smiling with your baby, and later playing social games with your toddler (such as "peekaboo" or "I'm going to get you"), are an important part of the development of this skill.

**Imitation** is also critical for speech and language learning. Children initially learn to imitate *your* imitation of *them,* and only later do they begin to imitate you directly or to invite you to play imitation games with them. For children who are learning language or learning how to make sounds and words, the prompts "look at me" or "watch this" are common ways we encourage a child to copy what he sees. It is also important to know that imitation of body movements is easier and comes before imitating words, sounds, and mouth movements.

We also consider the progression of **motor development**. In order for a child to develop his play skills, he must be able to move against gravity and hold himself upright. The development of the muscles in the trunk (or upper body) provides the freedom to then use his hands to manipulate toys and objects. This in turn allows him to experience the world visually and through the sense of touch and taste. In addition, the development of muscles in the trunk and ribcage allows for the mechanical production of sound and speech by expanding the amount of air he can use for making sounds. Bearing all of these skills in mind, we begin to see how many tasks must be accomplished before a child begins using words.

**Attention:** The second foundation skill that children must master is attention. When we think of attention, there are many words and concepts that come to mind. For our purposes, attention can be thought of as the ability to **select one thing to focus on out of all the possible things to focus on in the environment**. In addition, it is important to be able to *sustain that attention* so that you can get the benefit of that interaction, activity, or toy. As children get older, they're able to sustain for longer and longer periods and become better at weeding out distractions. A lot of concern is given to attention in the pre-academic years, and there's a lot of controversy over what children should be able to attend to and for how long. While it is not my purpose here to settle the argument, it is important to note that *attention has many facets and develops over a long period of time.* For our purposes, it is the quality of the attention and not just the length of it that is important. In addition, we must consider what kinds of activities result in sustained attention, and how readily children can transition from one focused activity to the next.

**Receptive Language/Understanding:** The next foundation skill children must master to become a confident communicator is the ability to understand what is being said. Children listen to language for nearly a year before they begin to use it, so it is important that they have not only the ability to tune in to language and listen actively but also to make sense of the language that is coming in and understand it. The ability to understand comes from a combination of listening skills, fund of knowledge/life experience, and processing and memory skills. As noted before, a child learns to associate words with the objects and actions he is experiencing.

**Play Skills:** As we learned before, play skills are an important component in speech and language development. There are many types of play that develop at predictable ages and stages, each of which provides the child with another layer of cognitive and linguistic challenge. The importance of play cannot be underestimated and will be discussed further.

**Social Skills:** The development of social skills is another important component of communication development. At its core, this is the dynamic interaction of two or more people. From the time an infant is born, she is interacting in a social context. The tools that she uses include eye gaze, body posture, crying, muscle tone, and many others. As this child develops, she begins to use words, gestures, tone of voice, body position, facial expression, and many other means to express herself and to make things happen in her world. The tremendous explosion in the diagnosis of children on the autism spectrum reflects a particular challenge in this area. Children with autism have significant difficulty in utilizing the language they have in a social context. They often struggle to make and maintain eye contact and to use conventional means to express themselves. With communication, it is not enough to have words; you have to know how to use them.

**Self-Regulation:** The next foundation skill we will discuss in this chapter is self-regulation. This relates to a child's ability to regulate his state or mood. In infants, we think of this as how easily he falls asleep or how easily he transitions from being asleep to being awake, and his temperament. For toddlers and young children, this also relates to how they are able to tolerate frustration and how easily they can soothe themselves into sleep or after a tantrum. Self-regulation skills are a concrete reflection of how the brain is organized and how well it is functioning. Children who have difficulty with self-regulation are often considered challenging because they present with many behaviors that are difficult to manage, and they may have unpredictable moods that can turn on a dime. Self-regulation skills are also a reflection of sensory processing skills.

**Sensory Integration:** Based on the groundbreaking and visionary work of A. Jean Ayres, sensory integration relates to how we take information in from our senses and use that information to act in the world.[3] Many children who have speech and language issues also have deficits in sensory processing, so it is important to understand the relationship between the two. Right now, at the moment that you are reading this, your brain is taking in millions of pieces of information from all of your senses and determining which pieces of information are relevant to what you're doing while filtering out the rest. That information is sent to the parts of your brain that dictate how you move and speak in response to your environment. We all have a sensory system that operates in different ways and at different levels of efficiency, and that is constantly changing over time.

For example, consider how you felt when you woke up this morning. Would you say that you were feeling well rested, ready to take on the world? Or did you feel lethargic and need something like a cup of coffee or a run to really wake up? Or perhaps the alarm or a screaming child or some other sudden noise or incident launched you into your day before you were ready? Consider what happened next. Were you able to take a soothing warm shower; did you read the paper, grab a cup of coffee—perhaps the first of many? Think about the strategies that you use to move yourself through your day in a way that keeps you available for thinking and problem solving and all of the complex tasks that you complete in a day. Your understanding of your own nervous system, and what keeps you working well, has evolved over a long period of time. Many young children lack of this awareness and understanding. Further, they are often subject to events that are beyond their control, whether it be their schedule, uncooperative peers or siblings, or even the high demands in a preschool environment.

A child's nervous system constantly has to adjust to what happens to him throughout the day, just as we do; however, children lack the insight, and often the ability or possibility, to just get what they need to stay organized. *Sensory integration* considers how easily and well a child is able to do this. Some children are frequently over-aroused, meaning that their system is running too high and too fast. This means they may be frequently frustrated, angry, or upset and may lack the ability to calm themselves down. On the other end of the spectrum, a child who is underaroused is frequently lethargic and may appear withdrawn and tired. This child has a hard time getting up the energy to play, to move, to eat, or to interact. Neither end of the spectrum allows for the development of new skills, practice of previously learned skills, or very functional interaction. It is important that we stay in the middle range or what we call *just right level of arousal*.[4] Being in this range allows us to access all of our higher level thinking skills and to move safely and efficiently through the day, completing tasks as they come up. In children who have difficulty with sensory integration, it impacts many of the skills needed for speech and language development, including attention, listening skills, receptive language, expressive language, play skills, social interaction, and especially self-regulation. We'll talk more about sensory integration later, but it is important to understand it at this foundations stage so that you can bear it in mind as we talk about the complexity of development.

## II: STAGES OF SPEECH AND LANGUAGE DEVELOPMENT

In the following section, information about development in the first five years is reviewed. Within each age range, information about the goals of that stage, as well as typical skill development, is reviewed. This is followed by a list of red flags that might indicate the need for further investigation. Feel free to refer to the section that applies to your child.

**Birth to Six Months:** The first stage is between birth and six months. The primary goal of this period is to **establish bonding with caregivers and to establish cycles of engagement and mutual interaction**. It is important to note that babies are born wired to communicate and that learning can begin even before birth. Just as an infant learns to read her parent's faces and she learns about situations as she grows and develops, parents also learn to read the baby's cues from the beginning. The primary communication skills that develop during this time are:

- Orienting to voices: An infant can focus on her mother's face for short periods of time directly after birth. Over the first six months she learns to recognize familiar people and primary caregivers. This means that she will quiet when she hears a voice she knows.
- Infants also learn to make and sustain eye contact and develop a social smile by four months.
- Cooing: This is primarily composed of open vowel sounds that may last from one second to several seconds. Back-and-forth cooing (where you and your baby take turns making sounds) also happens during this stage and can be considered the precursor to

conversation, where each participant takes turns in cycles to vocalize and listen. (Cooing usually sounds like a single vowel, such as "oo" or "ah" or "ee," produced with rising and falling intonation and varied loudness over time.)

- Crying is the primary means of communicating during this stage, and parents learn quickly how to differentiate the messages in a baby's cries. Most parents can tell within a few weeks whether a child is crying to indicate hunger, pain, or fatigue and respond accordingly. This is a critical piece of that *mutual engagement, or being tuned in to one another*.

- During this stage, there is limited play with objects, as infants lack the gross and fine motor skills to manipulate objects. Babies will typically gum anything that's put near their mouth during this stage, which is a part of feeding development as well. This is because the experience of a variety of textures helps children discover more about their mouth and how it works and helps them prepare for more complex textures in their food. Children may also reach for or swat at objects or bang them together if they are close enough to see.

- By the end of this period, infants are developing many other skills, including:

  - beginning to recognize their name;
  - searching for a speaker;
  - responding to tone of voice;
  - beginning to take turns vocalizing, and coos and laughs.

**Red Flags in This Stage**: Although infants with no medical history will all probably look fairly typical during this phase, children who are born with any significant medical or neurological condition are at high risk for difficulties, even in infancy. Of particular concern are children born prematurely. In my work in the neonatal intensive care unit (NICU), I often worked with parents of infants who were just learning to take the bottle or breast, or who were struggling with the development of their feeding skills. Just as important as learning to successfully feed, infants and parents need to tune in to one another and read the nonverbal cues that are available so that they can adjust their style of communicating and be responsive to the infant's messages. This work with social emotional communication and bonding was critical in overcoming the risks of premature birth and helping parents feel successful in working with their child. Those feelings of empowerment, and confidence in handling a fragile newborn, also allow the infant to feel secure and cared for, setting the stage for many of the language prerequisites we discussed earlier.

It may be appropriate to seek a referral for evaluation if:

- Your infant has a diagnosed neurological or other condition.
- Your infant struggles with feeding (breast or bottle).
- Your infant has difficulty with sleep or seems moody and/or in pain.
- You feel unable to connect or bond with your baby.
- Your baby does not smile or laugh or engage in eye contact.
- Your baby has limited interest in toys or interaction.

**Six to Twelve Months:** The second stage of language development is between six and twelve months. The primary goal of this stage is the **development of intention** and all of the prerequisite skills discussed earlier. In addition, first words typically occur during this period. The communication skills that develop during this stage are:

- Participation in social games such as peekaboo or "I'm going to get you." The development of anticipation also happens during this stage.
- Babbling and back-and-forth vocal play become more complex at this stage. Children go from producing mostly vowel sounds ("oo" and "ee") to producing consonants and vowels, alone or in combination with each other ("baba," "geegee," "haaaa"). Children often babble sounds made at the back of the mouth ("gaga," "keekee") and gradually add sounds made toward the front of the mouth ("baba," "mamamama," "dadada"). This back-and-forth vocal play is an important part of developing the speech sounds of a child's sound system; it also lays the foundation for the development of words that emerge later.
- Children at this stage begin to understand the word *no*, although they primarily respond to facial expression and tone of voice initially. You may see them stop what they are doing briefly, or they may cry when told "no" in a stern voice.

- Play at this stage consist primarily of putting toys in the mouth, banging and shaking toys, and dumping things out. Toward the end of the first year, children begin to engage in cause-and-effect play, such as pulling a string to get a toy, pop-ups, and push toys. This kind of play teaches children about doing something to get a predictable result.
- During this stage, many gestures develop, including pointing, waving, pushing away, lifting arms up to be picked up, head shakes, and high-fives. These gestures expand the range of what children are able to communicate, even if they don't have the words yet. Any child who learns to point vastly expands her world, since pointing can be used to request ("I want that."), or to label ("See that."), or to comment ("Look at that!").
- Children at this stage typically respond to their name, first by stopping what they're doing and later by turning to find the speakers voice.
- Children have an increased awareness of and interest in sound at the stage. They may indicate their wish to know what sounds are (truck, airplane doorbell, telephone) by showing they hear those sounds.
- During this stage, motor development occurs rapidly with the acquisition of rolling, sitting, crawling, and sometimes pulling himself up by holding onto you or the furniture. This increase in mobility frees up the hands to play with toys and to explore the world beyond what can be reached while sitting. Play skills increase in complexity and variety during this stage to include social games like peekaboo and filling and dumping.
- Other skills that develop during this stage:

  - recognizing the names of familiar people.
  - waving bye-bye, putting arms up to be picked up, pointing.
  - responding to simple questions and directions ("come here").
  - vocalization including *multisyllable* babbling ("babababa") and using the voice to get attention/greet and protest.
  - playing social games like "peekaboo!"
  - increased interest in words, and association of words and objects.

- beginning to identify body parts on request ("Where are your toes?").
- giving an object on request ("Give me the cup, please.").
- saying first words ("mama," "dada," "cookie," "up").
- beginning to use vocalization and gestures together to try to make things happen (saying "bye-bye" while waving).

**Red Flags**: During this stage, a lot is happening "behind the scenes," so to speak. Children are focused on learning strategies and in developing the intentions, or a clear objective for what he wants others to do. This can include getting a desired object, protesting a food he does not like, initiating a game, getting someone's attention, or refusing an unwanted toy. If you see the following kinds of behaviors, you may want to seek a screening or evaluation from an SLP:

- Unclear intent: Children are mimes in this stage; they use *everything* they have to make themselves understood, even when they only have a few words. If your child never seems to know what he wants, that warrants concern. This is also true if it seems that you know what he wants, but when he gets it, he still becomes upset.
- Infrequent attempts to communicate: Children at this stage are active in every way, learning to move and play and communicate. If your child seems withdrawn and does not respond to your attempts to play, or if he has limited reasons why he communicates, he may be having trouble with hearing or understanding the world.
- Limited sound play: Babies make noise! They cry and gurgle and coo and then babble. When babies are very quiet, this is unusual and may be a sign of something more serious, such as a hearing loss or significant speech disorder.

**Twelve to Twenty-Four Months:** The next stage in speech language development occurs between twelve and twenty-four months. The primary goal of this stage is to **increase vocabulary** by adding words to their repertoire, **to expand the reasons why they communicate** (from simply regulating the behavior of others to interacting for purely social purposes), and finally to **establish repair strategies** in the event that an initial attempt to communicate something is unsuccessful. During this stage, children may add up to one new word per week, but the development of single words is often uneven and unpredictable. I often speak with parents about the concept of vocabulary collected in a "leaky bucket." When a child adds a new word, he will frequently lose one that he had been using. This process of adding words and losing words and having them reappear is typical and reflects the tremendous changes that are happening across developmental systems. It is important to note as well that children in this stage are often very focused on their motor development. Because both communication development and motor development take a tremendous amount of cognitive resources, it is not uncommon to see your child become quieter as she focuses on her motor skills, only to become more verbal again once she has mastered walking. Understanding this helps to alleviate some concern that happens when children suddenly become less focused on verbal skills. In addition, we want to see children move through the various tasks that happen in this stage with the least amount of frustration possible. Some of the skills that develop during this time include:

- Children are able to more consistently follow simple commands ("sit down," "come here," "give it to me," "put it in," "no," and "stop.")
- By twenty-four months, children should have at least fifty words in their repertoire, but they may have as many as two hundred. Many times, children use a combination of *true single words* (remember how a real word was defined as one or more sounds used to reference something specific) combined with babbling to tell stories or try to express more complex thoughts. This is called *jargon*, and it is a true stage of development that should be celebrated. This stage can often look and sound like your child speaking a foreign language since they often use gestures and have the intonation of connected speech, but with only a few real words.
- Children are able to indicate "more," "all gone," and "all done."
- Children can answer simple *what* questions when asked for a label, provided that word is within their vocabulary ("What's this?").
- Imitation skills get stronger and more consistent during this time and become a viable learning strategy; this sometimes includes inconsistency in saying words on demand.

- Children are able to identify several body parts (on themselves or a doll) as well as common objects and familiar people (" mama," "dada," "cookie," "book," "teddy," "Auntie").
- Children begin to use gestures for indicating "yes" and "no." It is important to note that many children typically use one of these for both yes and no initially, which can lead to frustration when they say *no* but they really mean *yes*.
- There is a major expansion of play skills during this period with the development of *representational* play, (feeding, brushing, hugging dolls) and *pretend* play that reflects things they are familiar with, such as feeding a doll or giving a bath. They also become more able to do turn-taking activities, like rolling a ball back and forth with a partner. Constructive play also emerges in this stage, with skills such as stacking blocks and completing puzzles. Some children also enjoy imitating things they see you doing, such as talking on the phone, sweeping, or running the vacuum.
- Comprehension and understanding expand significantly during the stage and are critical to building vocabulary. Children at this stage continue to add new words, for body parts, people, and familiar songs. They also begin to understand action and spatial words (*in*, *on*, *next to*) and to follow more directions ("go get your shoes" and "throw that away").
- Somewhere between eighteen and twenty-two months, children often experience what is called a *lexical burst*. This is when they begin to express all of the words that they have understood for many months. This is an exciting time for both the child and family, as it seems as though they are developing many new words in a short period of time. For the child, this is when she truly begins to see how words are powerful because when she uses them, things happen. She can make an adult do or say or give her something that she wants. It is also during this period that the child may often learn that words are the most efficient way to get what they want, which is an important part of social communication development.
- Once children have about fifty words, they begin to combine them in short phrases. The chapter on language development has more in-depth information on this.
- Other skills that develop during this time are:

- using more words than gestures;
- asking, "What's that?" to get you to label an object;
- more consistent labeling of objects;
- an increase in the sounds that are produced correctly (/m/, /t/, /d/, /n/, /h/);
- some children beginning to call themselves by name or to use pronouns such as I/me.

**Red Flags**: During this stage, a lot is happening simultaneously so it can be difficult to determine whether a problem truly exists or not. Some behaviors that may indicate you need to seek an evaluation with an SLP:

- Difficulty adding words to vocabulary, or a steady loss of words that were mastered; this is different from the "leaky bucket" example in that a child with a more serious issue will lose words that have been consistently in his vocabulary, and usually this is seen after the tendency to drop words when new ones are learned has passed.
- Difficulty with or lack of imitation skills, meaning your child can't reproduce a movement or sound you have modeled.
- Difficulty answering simple questions or following directions, meaning that he does not respond at all, looks confused, or responds incorrectly.
- Frequent frustration and significant tantrums, especially when there is an expectation for communication.
- Overreliance on gestures and pantomime to get their point across, without babbling or development of words, especially after eighteen months; words should be steadily increasing by then.
- Limited development of sounds and limited use of vocalization, meaning he uses only vowel sounds ("ah" and "uh," rather than many different sounds).
- Feeding issues, such as difficulty with the movement of the muscles in the mouth and throat for swallowing, or difficulty accepting new foods and textures.
- Frequent allergies, ear infections, or snoring, as this may indicate possible hearing loss or other upper respiratory issues that impact speech development.

- Dependence on one person (usually Mom) to be the interpreter when he should be showing more independence. This can also look like a serious separation issue, since being away from you makes your child feel vulnerable.
- Reliance on structure and repetition, and difficulty managing change. This is a tricky one because all children at this age resist adult direction. They like to hear the same story over and over, or watch the same video, and they truly embody living in the moment. For this child, nothing could possibly be as good as what I am doing right now. This becomes a source of concern when redirection and artful dodging cannot move your child to comply. When tantrums are the norm rather than the exception, you may be looking at difficulties that go beyond typical toddler terrors.

**Two to Three Years:** The next stage in speech and language development occurs between two and three years. The primary goals of this stage include **the expansion of form, quantity, and complexity of spoken words, the significant expansion of the sound system and increased social awareness and interaction.** The primary skills that develop during this time are:

- A significant expansion in the richness and complexity of play to include more *dramatic play* (pretending to be a dinosaur), *pretend play* (playing house or kitchen) and *symbolic play* (being able to use a block as a phone or a tissue as a blanket; sequencing events in play, early games).
- Children are able to ask and answer basic *who*, *what*, and *where* questions ("Where's daddy?" "What's that?" and "Who is here?").
- Children are able to begin to combine two and three words to communicate for a variety of purposes such as requesting ("ant milk"), commenting ("the plane!"), labeling ("cookie," "ball"), calling ("Daddy!"), protesting ("No socks!") and negating ("Not your turn!" and "No, mine!").
- Vocabulary jumps to three hundred words during this stage and includes objects, actions ("clap," "kiss," "jump") and descriptor words ("hot," "sticky," "yucky," "blue").

- Children begin to develop syntax, including the use of plural *s* ("socks," "horses") and the present progressive "-ing" ("kicking ball," "eating apple").
- Children are able to match colors and shapes, even if they cannot label them ("blue," "green," and "yellow").
- There is a rapid increase in the level of clarity (for familiar listeners) in a child's speech from about 50 percent of his words at age two to about 75 percent of his words at age three; children have typically mastered the following sounds: /m/, /p/, /h/, /w/, /n/ by this time for words such as "my," "pop," "water," and "no."
- Other skills include:

  - Increase in the use of imitation as a way to learn new words (they often become like parrots at this stage, repeating everything they hear, even words you might not want them to say!).
  - Understanding size concepts and "one" and "all." ("Give me one block, please." and "Put all your Legos away in the bucket.")
  - Understanding the function of objects (that scissors cut and a broom sweeps) and part-whole relationships ("Show me the pedal on the bike, or the home button on the iPhone").
  - Greeting more consistently and without prompting, especially for people he knows well.
  - Answering *wh* questions and yes/no questions more consistently ("Where are your shoes?" and "Who broke this truck?").
  - Beginning to count from one to three with lots of modeling and help.

**Red Flags**: For toddlers, life is often frustrating. As your child is learning to balance her wants and needs with rules and what is expected of her, conflicts happen. She wants to explore and to be in control, but she often has to go without what she wants. It can be especially difficult at this stage to determine when behavior becomes concerning enough to get a consultation with an SLP, but here are some points to consider:

- Continued difficulty with adding/building vocabulary, meaning that your child uses a few words over and over and seems to have trouble learning new words, or if your child has trouble finding the right word, perhaps saying "dog" instead of "horse" or "bouncy thing" instead of "ball." In fact, some children rarely use specific words at all, preferring the more generic "thing" or "that."

- Difficulty in learning to combine words, so he stays stuck in the one-word phase, beyond what would be expected.
- Difficulty expressing ideas, or being unclear, meaning that your child just has difficulty in expressing herself overall, and she seems lost or confused when trying to tell you something. There can also be difficulty in telling you about something that happened when you were not there, such as in school. It is hard to follow the thread of what happened, and everyone is frustrated.
- Using words incorrectly, as described above.
- Continued difficulty with answering *wh* questions, or in asking them, meaning that he does not phrase questions appropriately ("Who that?" rather than "Who is that?" and "Where go mama?" rather than "Where did mama go?"), or he does not seem to know how to answer questions.
- Difficulty with play with toys, lack of interest in social interaction. Play is a social activity, so it is concerning if your child prefers to play alone and engages in repetitive play such as lining toys up, to the exclusion of any other kind of play.
- Significantly unclear speech, or few sounds used in words.
- Drooling or other feeding issues, which may indicate a problem with the muscles in the mouth.
- Difficulty sustaining attention to even favored activities, which may indicate many things, including the presence of fluid in the ears or a sensory challenge.

**Three to Four Years:** The next stage of language development occurs between three and four years and includes the following primary goals: to **increase the complexity of sentences** and **the complexity of play**, to **increase the content and meaning of language**, and **to increase clarity of speech.** The primary skills that develop during this period are:

- improved consistency with naming colors and shapes;

- use of three to four words together with grammatical constructs (plural, possessive, verb tense, -ing) for a range of reasons (requesting, greeting, calling, protesting, commenting, etc.);
- improved ability to follow two- to three-step commands ("Get your shoes and come downstairs" and "Put your book away and then clean up your toys");
- significant vocabulary growth, up to eight hundred to one thousand words, including object labels, actions, names of people, items in categories (animals), and descriptive words;
- mastery of /b/, /d/, /k/, /g/, /f/, the sounds in words like "baby," "doggie," "kiss," "go," and "fish."

**Red Flags**: During this stage, a child becomes more sophisticated in her use of language and her ability to interact with and control her world. Any of the following may be signs that there is a problem:

- Difficulty with increasing the length and complexity of sentences or staying stuck with short phrases.
- Difficulty finding the right words (she might say "cow" when she means "dog," or "heart" when she means "hot").
- Difficulty with answering and asking questions or telling about remote events (telling you about her day).
- Difficulty staying on topic, meaning that you may start out talking about the zoo, but suddenly she is talking about your family dog.
- Limited sounds or poor clarity of speech; if your child is difficult to understand at this age, there is a problem. Although some sounds develop much later (/r/, /th/), you should be able to understand your child about 90 percent of the time by age four.
- Appearing frustrated or withdrawn and avoiding communication. If your child does not enjoy talking and communicating and telling stories, or if she seems anxious whenever there is an expectation to use words, she may be having difficulty with understanding what she hears, expressing herself, or both.
- Poor listening or attention skills, difficulty following directions or remembering directions and events. Children are active, that is the reality. However, when you watch your child, you know if he seems to "get" what is going on and is perhaps a bit active, versus

seeing your child look confused by even routine activities he often does; that may signal a problem.

**Four to Five Years:** The next stage in speech language development occurs between four and five years. The primary goals of this stage include **increased use of language for mastering pre-academic skills** (such as counting, labeling letters, and following more complex directions). In addition, relationships become much more critical during this phase as does the social use of language. This includes negotiation with peers and *pretend* play. The primary skills that develop during the stage are:

- Rapid expansion of the pre-academic skills, including vocabulary, understanding concept development including spatial concepts (on, behind, above), size concepts (big, little, long, wide), and linguistic concepts ("comparing" words like *bigger* and *quieter*).
- Improved ability to follow up to three-step commands ("Put your backpack away, get a snack, and meet me at the car").
- More frequent production of sentences using four to seven words to communicate for a range of reasons.
- Improved ability to talk about remote events (I call this being "in the flow of time" as opposed to bound to the context of this moment).
- Use of pronouns (your, our, we, their, his, her) and modal verbs (can, should) develops.
- Significant increases in *imaginative* and *dramatic* play (playing dress-up, acting like superheroes).
- The development of narrative skills, which include the ability to create and recall stories and events according to the framework of storytelling.
- Speech development is largely accomplished except for later developing sounds and consonant blends. Clarity of speech should be near 100 percent in conversation, at least for familiar listeners. Additional sounds mastered at this age include: /s/, /sh/, /j/, /ch/, /z/, /v/, /l/ for words like "sun," "shoe," "jump," "zoo," "van," and "lamb."

**Red Flags:** Most children who have a difficulty will have already been identified by this age, but here are some signs that a concerning behavior may need further investigation by an SLP:

- difficulty with clarity of speech and not mastering sounds;
- difficulty with forming sentences, especially if there are issues with word order or grammar;
- difficulty understanding directions or questions, or seeming lost or one step behind in activities;
- limited communication for social purposes, or restricted play;
- lack of flexibility or needing control in play or daily routines;
- difficulty tolerating changes to the routine, or transitions.

## III: SUPPORTING SPEECH AND LANGUAGE DEVELOPMENT

The next section will discuss how to support the development of speech and language in young children. This is by no means an exhaustive discussion but should provide some basic principles and ideas that can be a bridge until you are able to access some direct intervention.

### Myths of Language Development

Below are five common myths about language development. These "conventional wisdoms" represent some of the most common mistakes that people can make in trying to help kids learn to communicate. Understanding the truth behind these myths gives you knowledge and direction in how to direct your efforts toward communication development in the most effective ways.

**MYTH 1: Children need to be taught language.** Although the focus of this book is on what happens when something goes wrong, for children who are typically developing, language unfolds in an easy and natural way. Language naturally follows from *experience*, and children learn many things by watching others and participating in events. Language is not learned through flashcards and artificial experiences with technology, no matter how educational those toys or programs claim to be. There is no substitute for natural experience, whether that be a trip to the zoo or setting the table at home. While it may be true that some children in speech and language therapy are given structured tasks and more contrived activities to practice a specific skill such as a target speech sound, the primary focus should be on *doing* and interacting in a more natural way with objects and experiences.

**MYTH 2: All children learn language the same way.** There are at least two distinct types of language learners, and understanding a child's style is helpful in directing strategies to his language and play. Some children learn easily by listening and seem to pick words up quickly after a single exposure. This type of language learner actively adds words to his vocabulary, easily moves through the stages of development, and seems to progress in a linear way. In contrast, a different style might mean a child learns more by watching and seems to lean toward being on the sidelines. This type of style often means learning language more slowly, often adding phrases or chunks of language at a time. This child is a more hesitant communicator and needs more repetition and modeling before he will try something on his own. Knowing your child's style will help you to match your strategies to his needs and modify how you model language and communication in ways that suit him best.

**MYTH 3: Complex toys are better than simple old school toys.** As any parent knows, the boom in electronics and talking toys is hard to resist; however, the usefulness of these toys is often limited. In my experience, the novelty of these toys wears off quickly, and the child is usually drawn to the electronic aspect of the toy to the exclusion of actually learning to play. We want to encourage appropriate play, but also creativity and flexibility with toys. Using toys with a lot of electronics often encourages isolation and discourages problem solving and creativity. In my office, I even removed the batteries from my Fisher Price Farm set because I wanted the kids to make their own animal sounds! This is not to imply that technology has no value, especially with children who struggle to communicate, but rather that it has become out of balance. We want to be sure we are providing language-rich opportunities along with developing the skills to use technology, which is its own form of literacy. If you have ever had the experience of a young child being more excited about the box a toy comes in than the toy itself, you can appreciate the truth behind this myth. Almost *anything* can be a toy, and part of the development of play skills involves using the imagination to turn ordinary objects into fanciful pieces of wonder. This is how a wrapping-paper tube becomes a sword, or an ordinary tissue becomes a magical cape for a superhero.

**MYTH 4: Children learn from toys alone**. Play is an interactive sport, and toys represent a context ripe with opportunities for interaction. From infancy, children learn to associate words with objects and actions they experience by hearing the word while looking at or using an object. Meaning is learned by the processing of words and feeling attached to the things they are doing. Many children, especially those who have developmental challenges, need to be shown how to interact with toys, and how to expand play from throwing or banging toys to more sophisticated play. This is often overlooked when it is assumed that kids will just *know* how to use a toy and that limitations in their play skills are really just their preference. Play is the context where children learn that activities have a beginning and an end, that there are goals to be met, and how to transition between activities. Parents, and even siblings, can help to model these skills for children, using positive strategies to support development and expansion of play. In a follow-up to Myth 3, electronics and other talking technologies do not possess the aspects of child-directed stimulation that guide each little one to success and problem solving, helping her learn to navigate her world.

**MYTH 5: All language input is created equal**. If this were true, no one would need the specialized services of a speech language pathologist, since everyone would know what to do and how to do it! There are things that we have learned from research and clinical experience that show us how children learn best; this is true for typically developing children and those with challenges. In the remaining pages of this chapter, you will take your first steps to becoming a wise and successful facilitator, coach, and model. It is a powerful and noble thing to help a child learn to express himself effectively and independently. In many cases, making slight adjustments in how you interact with your child can go a long way to helping him get to where he needs to be. For other children, the process may be longer, and more complex. Rest assured, however, that SLPs are well equipped to help you and your child move through this process as successfully as possible.

There are many ways to support your child in learning to listen, talk, and communicate. One of the most important aspects to consider is **how the environment the child is in creates (or hinders) opportu-**

**nities for communicating.** There are a few areas that consistently come up in my work with families:

*Problem: Toys that are too accessible/too many toys.* Children these days have access to a wide variety of toys, from cars and trucks to train tables, mountains of puzzles, and books, as well as all kinds of electronics. In many homes, children's toys have taken over rooms of the house, and nothing is organized. There are often missing pieces and broken toys strewn everywhere, and children play as they will, with no structure. This often results in complaints about how children never stay with anything very long, and they often take multiple toys out without cleaning up.

*Solution*: Limit the toys that are accessible at any one time. While is it great to have toys that kids can access and play with on their own, *your child will need to be taught organizational strategies.* He does not know how to manage his toys, or how to structure play so that each activity has an ending that includes cleaning up. In addition, when a child has too many choices, he will often skim the surface of playing and never go deeply enough to really benefit from the language opportunities available with that activity. Using boxes or clear bins and storing similar toys together can be very helpful. You can then use pictures of the toys (bin for puzzles, bin for blocks, bin for cars) to create a picture board or book that encourages your child to request things from you. The requirement that your child clean up one activity before moving on to something else helps to tame the chaos and keeps things together.

*Problem: I only want my cars and trucks.* Your child may want to play with the same toys over and over and ignore the rest or just throw them around. This is related to the issue above, and can be a function of simple overwhelm, boredom, or lack of understanding about how to use toys. I often see children who need modeling and explanation about how to use toys; it is not always intuitive.

*Solution*: Rotate toys weekly. You can use a theme (animals, vehicles, sensory play) and just have toys related to that theme available that week. This will allow you to really play with your child and her toys, for her to learn about vocabulary and concepts that are related to the theme. At the end of that week, bring out a new set of toys; it will feel special to your child because novelty draws children back in! Even if they are toys that he has had for a long time, they will feel new, and he is more likely to engage with those toys. Play with your child so he can see how to use that toy. Take turns, and talk about what you are doing, so he develops a solid understanding.

*Problem*: *Tantrum tantrum tantrum!* Your child uses grunting, pointing, throwing, and screaming to try to get what he wants, and everyone is frustrated. This happens a lot when kids are slow to develop words, or when they are the type to stubbornly refuse to use the words they have. Children learn quickly who will "fill in the blanks" and give them what they want without the effort of saying, or trying to say, words. This can become a vicious cycle, one that slows their development overall and can leave you as the parent feeling like nothing is progressing. In some cases, children may have genuine difficulty moving forward, but in any case, it is important to *create* opportunities for communication.

*Solution*: *Wait*. Let your child come to you to request help, or for an object. When he uses a tired strategy like screaming, ask him to tell you what he wants. Encourage him to say a sound, use a sign, or imitate the word—whatever is at least slightly beyond what he is doing now. Offer choices, such as, "Do you want _____ or _____?" and allow him to tell you what he wants. Use pictures and choice boards to encourage him to be more independent in making choices. Above all, refuse to fill in the blanks just because you know what he wants. Sometimes your child has to get frustrated enough to bridge the gap and leap into using words.

*Problem*: *Your child won't play with you, and he doesn't listen—he just runs around*. Children have short attention spans, especially when they are toddlers. They like to explore, to crash, and to knock things over. They focus on the action and the fun, they don't often listen to lots of complicated sentences or directions, and they don't often answer questions in play. I often see parents use "test questions" such as, "What color is this block?" and "How many crayons do you have?" in an attempt to engage the child. These questions have nothing to do with the play that is happening, and kids are sensitive to the perceived demands of empty questions, resulting in a lack of response.

*Solution*: *Meet her where she is*. Sink into her play, and follow her lead. Talk about what she is doing, looking at, interacting with. And keep your language related to her play. Leave the questions for the true opportunities where you need to decide together where the play will go next. Questions like, "What should we do now?" and "What do you want

for lunch?" are true questions that maintain the flow of your communication.

## Types of Language Stimulation

Let's discuss some different types of language stimulation that you can
use when playing with your child. There are two primary types of language stimulation—*direct* and *indirect.*

**Direct language stimulation** is adult focused and uses primarily
questions and directives, telling a child what to do and how to do it. As
discussed above, many children are sensitive to demands and do not
respond well to this type of play. They lose interest quickly because it
does not engage their interests and it feels forced and constrained.

In contrast, **indirect language stimulation** is child focused and
creative. It is designed to capitalize on your child's attention and his
discoveries, giving voice and shape to his internal dialogue, and showing
him the way to play. This helps him to understand and use the language
that goes with his play. There are several distinct types of indirect
language stimulation:

- Self-Talk: This is simply talking about what you are doing, as you
  do it. This lends itself well to daily routines, as well as activities
  with a sequence of steps. If you are washing your hands, you talk
  about how you are turning on the water, rubbing in the soap, and
  making bubbles. You talk about how you rinse your hands and dry
  them with a towel. This is especially useful when your child is
  helping you or shadowing you in an activity. Self-talk helps children learn the vocabulary and sequence of things, and it is very
  natural and easy.
- Description: This is similar to "parallel talk" (see below), but it
  focuses on what the child is doing. You might talk about how they
  are pushing the car "up up up the ramp . . . now let it go!" It goes
  down the ramp and around the track. Or you might talk about
  pouring the tea in the cups, adding some milk, stirring the tea,
  and having a sip. It allows the child to take the lead because you
  are just wrapping the language around the activity and not directing it.

- Parallel talk: This technique allows you to narrate *your* play with the child. "My monkey is climbing the tree . . . he loves to grab the bananas. MMMMM, he has three bananas! Look, he can peel the banana and chomp chomp chomp! He is eating all the bananas. OOH OOH, I'm all done bananas—time for a nap!" Again, it is focused on the play and shows your child how to construct a play theme and follow it through, without directing her to do anything specific. Chances are, if you have her attention, she will probably copy what you do.

- Expansion: This technique is useful for a child who is working on moving from single words to combinations, or from two words to longer sentences. Whatever your child says, you *expand* it by adding an element. For example, if your child says "car" while pushing a car, you can say, "Yes, the blue car" or "That car goes fast!" This shows your child how to expand the complexity and meaning of his message, but without a demand for production or imitation.

- Expansion plus correction: This technique is useful for a child who is working on saying longer sentences and needs support to expand the form. If your child says "Car goed up and over," you can respond with, "Yes, the car *went* up and over the hill." You are adding to the message and making a subtle correction, again, without the expectation of performance. The key is to *validate the message (content) but model the more sophisticated form.*

### General Language Stimulation Strategies

Here are some additional general language strategies that may be helpful in supporting your child as she begins to acquire language:

- Limit the complexity of your language. This is especially important for a child at the earliest stages of language development. While it is tempting to want to provide rich, complex sentences, he cannot imitate you at that level. It is much more useful to match your language with the level that he is currently at; if a child is at the single-word level, we use single words. If he is trying to use two words together, we use mostly single- and two-word combinations.

- Rephrase and repeat. Don't be afraid to use a single word multiple times—"up up up"—or to modify as sentence to be only slightly different ("I am going up the ramp; let's go up"). This relates to limiting the complexity of your language and greatly helps your child to understand and, hopefully, imitate what you have said.
- Be on your child's level. Sit down to play or kneel down to talk, and make sure that you have his attention before speaking. Sometimes it is also helpful to hold an object by your mouth or eyes to focus his attention to your face before you speak. This kind of visual contact primes him for hearing and processing what you are going to say.
- Be consistent with daily routines. Language is happening all the time, in all the activities that we do every day with children, such as bathing, dressing, feeding, and playing. The language that we use in these activities tends to be consistent and can help greatly with learning vocabulary concepts and sequencing. Daily routines are wonderful opportunity to teach your toddler in a very natural way.
- Limit distractions. When you take time for quality play with your child, try to eliminate excessive background noise and other distractions. Turn off the TV, keep the music soft, and make it a time for you to focus on each other.
- Expand on your child's interests and follow his lead. We have discussed this before. Your child is more likely to tune in, pay attention, and stay with you and perhaps even imitate your words when what is being said relates to what he is doing, playing with, thinking about, or looking at. Let your child lead you in play.
- Validate the attempt and encourage imitation. This relates to the concept of *validating content and modeling form*. Be proud of your child's attempts to say words and to interact with you. Let him know! And then show him the next level of language, using *expansion* or *correction*, two strategies that were discussed in an earlier section.
- Limit the use of test questions. This is one of *the most important strategies* you can learn if you are trying to encourage communication. Test questions have no place in this context. The use of real questions that solicit opinion or help to guide the play are

acceptable and natural. Questions that have no real relevance to the activity and only place demands on the child should be avoided. This is also true of using primarily yes/no questions that limit what a child can produce.

- Use *wait* time strategically. As parents, and loving adults, we don't want to see children struggle. And when we feel we know what she wants, it is tempting to jump in and provide the word, or just give her the object. This denies her the opportunity to push herself to try using a word or sign or other skill. When you present a choice, or ask a question, *wait*. Then wait some more. Sometimes a child can take twenty to thirty seconds to make an attempt to answer. Waiting gives her the space to try and lets her know you will not just jump in. It can be challenging at times, but this is one of the most important strategies I teach parents to use.

This chapter has provided a detailed look into the many aspects of speech and language development that happen in the first five years. It is quite an accomplishment when your child is able to navigate this complex web of intentions, structures, and interactions. For those children who have failed to develop language as expected, the strategies provided here are good ways to get started while you look into an evaluation with a speech language pathologist. There will be a more detailed review of that process in chapter 4.

# 4

# ASSESSMENT OF SPEECH AND LANGUAGE DISORDERS

There are many ways to reach the point of obtaining a comprehensive evaluation from a speech language pathologist (SLP), including initiating one on your own, or as a referral from your child's primary care physician, usually the pediatrician. What is most important, in my clinical experience, is to trust your instincts. If you feel that there is a problem, and you are concerned, continue to dialogue with your pediatrician until you are able to proceed with at least a consultation. If there is not a problem, your concerns will have been addressed, and you can move on. If there is a clinical problem, you won't spend precious time waiting and watching as the problem gets worse. In the case of communication skills, this usually shows up as frustration and difficult behaviors, which stem from an inability to express even basic wants and needs, and a continued dependence on you, at a time when your child's independence should be increasing.

When you speak to your pediatrician, it is important to share your concerns as completely as possible. Generally speaking, your child's speech and language skills will be screened at annual physicals and checkups. You may be asked how many words your child has, or how well he or she follows directions. While these are good basic questions that should be asked, your child's physician may not tap into your concerns about what is going on with your child. Be proactive in discussing how your child is developing as a communicator, including where there may be challenges or areas that don't seem to be going well. It is also helpful to have a reference for speech and language development to make the conversation more specific. One suggestion is to go the website for the American Speech Language Hearing Association, at Asha.org, to find printable resources for tracking the development of communication skills.

Physicians will sometimes encourage you to wait and see what happens to allow time for the natural variation in child development or for the impact of gross motor development on communication to ease. This is an unfortunate myth that still persists within some medical circles. The fact is that we *know* that there is a critical period of development in the first five years, with the years before age three being particularly critical for intervention to have the greatest impact on brain organization and development.[1] In addition, children who are progressing normally through developmental stages may have passing frustration, but their challenges are not front and center in everyday life. If your child is struggling with communication, it is important to identify it as early as possible so that he or she, and you, can get the help you need.

In 2016, there is a heightened awareness of autism spectrum disorder (ASD), a diagnosis that often includes lifelong medical and developmental challenges. There are programs and procedures in place to screen specifically for these disorders because they have become part of the fabric of physician awareness due to significant public awareness of this condition. Many parents who seek a screening or even an evaluation are afraid to find out if their child has autism, and will often ask about that as one of their first questions. While this is important, and I support such screenings, the fact that your child does not have signs and symptoms of ASD does not mean he does not have a problem. There are many other speech and language disorders that can occur, sometimes without an easily identifiable cause, that still require diagnosis and treatment.

Once you are able to reach consensus with your pediatrician, she can provide you with necessary referrals that may be required by your insurance carrier. She may also direct you to a specific agency or private speech pathology practice that your physician wants you to contact to set up an appointment. It is critical to be proactive in contacting your insurance company to verify eligibility and coverage for speech language pathology services. This information may include co-pays, deductibles, and co-insurance. You should also be aware of your out-ofpocket maximums and any conditions that are not covered by your health insurance plan. The member services department of your insurer can also tell you if you have a limited number of visits, whether a prescription or referral is required from your pediatrician, and when you will need to reauthorize your services after an initial period of treatment. In many cases, services may be covered if they meet the definition of "medical necessity," something that your speech-language pathologist will determine during the evaluation process. It is important to note that many plans will not cover conditions that are considered to be "developmental" and that might resolve on their own, but they will cover conditions that are the result of an accident or illness. The logic to this is that you can't rehabilitate something you never had (learning to talk versus regaining that ability after a stroke). There is currently a movement to require insurance companies to cover *habilitative* services, or those services that develop a skill that has not yet developed, but you should check with your plan to be sure.

Depending on the age of your child at the time of referral, you may be seen by different agencies or practitioners. If you begin services before the age of three years, you might be seen in an early intervention (EI) program, which is a federally mandated program administered by each state. These programs provide a variety of developmental and family support services, often in the home or natural environment, designed to help your child master skills within a developmental framework. Once you contact the EI program, there is a series of steps that are required in order to begin services. These steps include an initial intake, completing a developmental evaluation, and the drafting of an Individualized Family Service Plan (IFSP). This plan outlines your child's strengths and needs, her eligibility for services, and the functional outcomes you want your child to achieve. Once your child qualifies for services, based on the level and severity of the identified delays, he can participate in a variety of individual therapies, groups, and family services. He will be reevaluated at regular intervals, and the plan will be updated as needed.

When your child turns three, services are provided by the public schools, should they still be needed, according to the current federal laws regarding special education. If you have been receiving EI, your team of therapists and your family service coordinator (FSC) will participate in the transition to the schools and assist the educational team with the development of the Individualized Education Plan (IEP). If a referral is made to the public schools by an EI program, a team of educators and therapists in your local school district will evaluate your child again. The school-based team will use federally defined criteria to determine whether your child is eligible to receive services, based on how his disabilities will affect his ability to learn and socialize in a school setting. The results of your child's evaluations will be used to determine the type and intensity of services your child will need to succeed. This might include a classroom and/or specific therapies such as speech and occupational therapy (OT) or physical therapy (PT).

One of the decisions that needs to be made is whether your child can learn in a classroom that includes typical peers, called an *integrated classroom*, or if they need to be educated in a *substantially separate* classroom, where there are fewer children, usually with more intense needs. This can be a complex question to answer, due to the multiple factors that are at play within the classroom. This question also affects how much time your child may be pulled out of the classroom for therapy services versus having those services delivered in the classroom (inclusion). In fact, for some children, a public school placement won't be sufficient to meet their needs, and they may need to spend some time in a program with specialized training or programming, such as a school for the deaf and hard of hearing, or a school for those with autism spectrum disorder (ASD). It is advisable to spend some time going to and observing different kinds of programs that might work for your child in the months leading up to their third birthday. Your EI team should be able to provide you with recommendations that might be appropriate, and they can often go with you to visit and help you ask the right questions.

The transition from EI services to the public school can be a challenging one. While EI most often happens in your home, and you are an active participant in all sessions, this changes radically once your child goes to school. In almost all schools, your child must separate from you, and you are not directly involved in their classroom or therapy experiences. This can be a hard turn for parents, especially when your child can't communicate easily or well. It requires extra effort to build relationships with your child's teachers and therapists and to establish communication so that you are in the loop.

Qualifying for services through the public schools is very different from qualifying for EI, which can result in confusion. Children must exhibit a fairly significant deficit in order to be placed in a classroom at age three. If your child's difficulties are not severe enough to qualify for a classroom, she may be able to receive services on a "drop-in" basis at the school. This usually means that she has an isolated speech and language issue, but she does not require the additional support for education. In addition, the way services are delivered in the schools is different, too. Children who may have received a lot of one-to-one treatment in EI will begin participating in groups or treatment provided within the classroom. It is important to work with your school team to determine the best type and frequency of treatment for your child, taking into account all of your child's strengths and needs and their learning style.

In addition to these school-based services, you may be able to access an evaluation by going directly to a hospital, rehabilitation agency, or private SLP practice. Sometimes, you can even access a free screening, which would indicate whether an evaluation is needed. Again, it is important to understand what is covered by your health care plan and what you may be responsible for financially.

Once a referral for a speech language pathology evaluation is in place, you should contact the SLP or agency that you wish to use. You will need to complete an initial intake process, giving some basic information about your child, your concerns, and your insurance information. You will be asked about your availability, and an appointment will be booked. In most cases, you will be sent a comprehensive case history form to complete prior to your visit. This gathers much more detailed information about your child's birth, medical, developmental, and educational histories. In my practice, I usually have the parent bring the case history form back at the time of their visit. It is critically important that you complete the case-history form so that the major part of your child's appointment is spent focusing on him or her and conducting any necessary tests. When a case history form is not completed, valuable time has to be spent conducting an interview; that is time not spent with your child. Some of the information collected in the case history can give the SLP valuable information about such things as:

- your child's preferences and favorite activities;

- challenging behaviors and triggers;
- other SLP testing that may have already been done;
- medical or developmental events that indicate the need for referrals to other medical or therapeutic professionals;
- a general sense of how development is progressing by looking at how developmental milestones have been met and which have not been met.

At the time of your evaluation, you will likely be asked for a copy of your insurance card, the case history, and copies of other relevant documents. Depending on the setting and the SLP, you may be asked to accompany your child into the room for testing, or you may be asked to stay in the waiting area while your child goes in for testing. In my practice, I do not typically ask parents to separate from their child under the age of three years. I feel it is important for the child to feel comfortable in order for me to get the best picture of his or her skills. If you are asked to separate from your child, you may be able to watch the session through a one-way mirror. Be sure to speak with the SLP about any concerns you have about leaving your child. In my experience, some parents feel their child does better when they do separate because she relies heavily on mom or dad and may not engage with a stranger; other parents feel their child's anxiety at separation will override her ability to demonstrate her skills at all.

During the evaluation itself, the SLP has several primary tasks. First and foremost is to establish a rapport with your child. Kids who are afraid, or feeling anxious, will not perform well; in fact, they may say nothing at all. This initial period may involve playing, reading books, or doing some gross motor activities such as ball play or using a trampoline or tunnel that may help them feel at ease. The second task is to conduct testing that will provide the information necessary to reach a diagnosis, or at least a solid understanding of your child's profile. This may involve several elements:

- Formal, standardized testing. These are tools that we use that must be administered in a certain way, and they provide scores that allow comparison of your child's performance to others his age.

- Informal testing. This can include many different types of tests, including checklists, parent interview tools, guided play, or specific attempts to elicit a particular skill.
- Clinical observation. This is happening throughout the evaluation, from the time your child meets the SLP in the waiting room. This information provides the qualitative balance to the numbers obtained on formal testing and can be just as important as testing. It also includes documentation of behavior, including test-taking behavior, attention, and work ethic and how your child responds to the performance demands of testing.
- Feedback and wrap-up. This is an opportunity for the SLP to give you some preliminary impressions and to answer any questions you may have.

Once the evaluation is complete, the SLP must look at all the data and determine a diagnosis and a treatment plan. As part of this, SLPs consider formal test scores, informal testing information, behavior observations, parent concerns, and case history information. As SLPs, we also look at sensory factors and learning-style information in order to determine the best way to help your child. This may also include referrals to other professionals for further testing, such as to neuropsychologists, neurologists, audiologists, otorhinolaryngologists (ear, nose, and throat), or others. All the information is then put together in a clinical report that outlines the recommendation for services, as well as long- and short-term goals.

Most clinical reports have a similar framework, which is outlined below. The report is designed for several purposes, including: justifying medical necessity and defining disability for insurance companies for payment purposes; providing information to schools or EI team members about your child's communication profile; and educating you about how your child is developing and what his or her needs are. One of the challenges in doing this is to write the report at a level that makes sense to you as a parent while providing necessary information, which sometimes includes professional jargon intended for other health care practitioners who might read the report. One of the greatest compliments I receive is when a parent says to me, "This is exactly my child. You captured perfectly what is going on, and helped me to understand."

It is important that you understand what the report is saying so that you can begin to help your child in the therapeutic process. If you do not understand what something means, it is your responsibility to *ask* for clarification. It is the SLP's responsibility to help you learn about your child's communication and his or her difficulties, but we use professional jargon and "alphabet soup" all the time with colleagues in health care and education, and we sometimes forget that others do not know that specific vocabulary. I have seen many parents indicate nonverbally that they do not understand something but then not ask a question. If you do not know what is going on, you cannot be the advocate you need to be for your child.

## COMPONENTS OF AN EVALUATION REPORT

The following are common elements in most SLP reports, although they may vary in sequence; this list is not meant to be exhaustive. Depending on the specific concerns that are identified, your SLP may look at any and all of these areas.

- *Demographic information*: Your child's name, date of birth, date of evaluation, chronological or corrected age, referral source, diagnosis, and relevant diagnosis codes used by insurance companies.
- *Reason for referral*: A brief description of the reason the evaluation was conducted, including your primary concerns.
- *History information*: A complete review of the medical history (including pregnancy course and birth), developmental history, and educational history. This section will also identify current services, allergies, medications, and other service providers who see your child.
- *Behavioral observations*: This section includes general observations of your child's behavior during the evaluation, as well as test-taking behavior. It is common to indicate how reliable the results are as an indicator of your child's true abilities. Sensory issues, attention issues, and test anxiety may also be mentioned here, along with any strategies that seemed helpful in facilitating your child's participation.

- *Clinical results*: This includes all testing results from formal and informal testing, typically organized by topic area. Generally, there may be information on the following areas:

  - Oral motor skills—an assessment of the muscles in and around your child's mouth and how adequately they work to support speech and feeding skills. This may also include information about cranial nerve function, symmetry, and muscle tone and how your child is able to execute specific kinds of movement (rounding the lips or elevating the tongue) during speech and on demand.
  - Feeding skills—an assessment of how your child manages various textures, including liquids and different kinds of foods. We look at how your child uses his or her mouth to bite, chew, and swallow, as well as any behaviors that negatively impact feeding.
  - Articulation/sound production skills—this is more thoroughly addressed in chapter 5, but includes an assessment of the kinds of sounds your child makes in words and how easy it is to understand their speech.
  - Receptive language/processing/memory skills—this is covered in chapter 6, but may include a variety of tasks designed to look at your child's attention and listening skills, how easily they process information, and how they are able to recall what they have heard or read.
  - Expressive language skills—this is also covered in chapter 6, but may include a variety of tasks designed to look at how your child expresses him- or herself, including vocabulary, sentence complexity, and use of grammar, and the social context of how your child communicates.
  - Voice—an informal assessment of pitch, loudness, and vocal quality. We need to determine if there are any issues, such as hoarseness or loss of voice, that might indicate the need for a medical workup.
  - Fluency—an informal assessment of how your child produces *connected speech* and whether there are any concerns about stuttering. In young children, this also includes differ-

entiating between normal or developmental dysfluency and a developing stutter.

- Reading/writing skills—this may involve either formal or informal testing to determine how well your child is reading and writing. We look at components including spelling, generation of sentences, comprehension of written language, and organization and complexity of their writing.
- Phonological awareness/processing skills—this may involve formal or informal testing of your child's mastery of auditory-based pre-reading skills, including rhyming, blending sounds to words, breaking words down into syllables and sounds, and isolating sounds in words.
- Other—depending on the specific concerns, your SLP may also test/probe skills such as executive function, attention, narrative skills (story telling), and more.

It should be noted that not every evaluation requires all of these elements. For example, a child with an articulation disorder may not require extensive language testing. A child being seen for a voice disorder may not undergo formal articulation testing.

- *Clinical impressions/summary*: This section provides a unifying statement about your child's communication skills, including any diagnosis (if appropriate) and an assessment of severity for each area. A recommendation for/against therapy services is also seen here.
- *Recommendations*: This section has several components, including:

  - Frequency of intervention—where sessions will occur, for how long, and how many times per week;
  - Long-term goals—the primary goal that is being targeted. An example for expressive language would be that your child would be able to use complete, grammatical sentences to express him- or herself across a range of tasks. For an articulation disorder, the long-term goal might be that your child will be understood by unfamiliar listeners 85 percent of the time, across situations.

- Short-term goals/objectives—this will include the target skill, accuracy level, prompts, and cues required. These are the smaller steps needed to achieve the long-term goal. For the expressive language goal identified above, one short-term objective might be that your child can use complete sentences when requesting help or in describing objects. A short-term goal for the child with the articulation deficits above might be that she will use a target sound in all positions within words at the sentence level. It provides more specific information about what your child needs to be working on *right now.*

- Strategies, accommodations, and parent/educator training—information about any specific strategies that will be used, or areas where you as the parent may need some specific instruction in order to support your child's achievement of short-term goals.

- Referrals to other professionals as needed—any specific concerns will be discussed here. Examples might include referral to an audiologist for a complete hearing test, or to a neuropsychologist for more detailed information about cognitive skills and educational planning.

- Prognosis and target for reevaluation—a statement about the expectation for progress with the recommended intervention, and when testing should be conducted again. This is typically in six or twelve months, although it may be shorter for children with mild difficulties where progress is expected to be rapid.

- Closing statement and signature, with the provider's credentials.

SLPs must determine what functional deficits exist and develop a plan to maximize communication effectiveness. This should include both your goals as a parent and clinically driven goals, based on the developmental framework or an understanding of any limitations indicated by your child's diagnosis. For very young children, we want to focus on helping them achieve developmental milestones as much as possible, following the typical progression as closely as we can. For older children, we may focus on filling in the gaps or providing compensatory strategies that allow the child to keep up with social or academic demands while we work on developing those specific skills that are deficient. For children who are more medically or neurologically involved, we focus on maximizing opportunities for communication and developing a total communication system that allows them to interact successfully with their environment, while developing specific speech and language skills.

Depending on where you have your initial evaluation, and whether treatment is recommended, you may receive services according to one of many models. This may include one primary or many professionals working together to help you and your child. In addition, as mentioned above, you may be working within a medical model (through a hospital or agency) or through the public schools. For the best of both worlds, working with a private-practice SLP may be a good option for you. In my practice, I use the medical and developmental models together, looking at the whole child and the family. This allows me to provide direct and indirect support for clinically driven and family-driven goals, while also taking into account the educational needs of the child.

It is likely that your child will have more than one area of difficulty in terms of speech and language, and your SLP will be tasked with providing the most effective treatment. This may include a direct teaching approach, where you and/or your child are being taught something specific. Examples of this include learning where your tongue goes to make a particular sound, learning a strategy for remembering what you have heard, or learning how to ask a *wh* question. There may be highly structured activities that provide specific and repetitive opportunities for your child to practice the new skill with prompts and cues. In contrast, your child's speech and language sessions may also include experiential activities, where your child is being guided through a learning opportunity with more informal supports in place. This encourages incidental learning, or learning by doing. This may also include opportunities to practice a learned skill that is now being generalized beyond a highly structured activity. These kinds of activities may also include more motor and sensory components, and may be more motivating to your child. It is important to remember, however, that *both* types of activities will likely be required during your child's treatment. We have to learn something before we can practice it, and we have to practice it before we can generalize it, and we have to generalize it before it becomes automatic.

Completing an initial SLP evaluation can take from days to months, depending on how long you have to wait for an appointment. Coming to the decision where you feel an evaluation is necessary is also a process that takes some time. Once you determine that you want to look deeper at your child's communication, take the time to educate yourself about speech and language development. Engage in active dialogue with your pediatrician about your concerns, and ask for a referral. Don't be satisfied to wait and see while the clock ticks and time goes by. Getting a qualified SLP on your team can be miraculous for your child, and it can make a huge difference in his or her life, and in yours.

# 5

# AN OVERVIEW OF SPEECH SOUND DISORDERS

As you may recall from chapter 2, *speech* is the act of producing sounds for verbal communication. This chapter will discuss children who have difficulty with this, earning a diagnosis related to speech sound production (articulation). This category of disorders would also include issues with voice production and fluency (stuttering); these are broad topics and are beyond the scope of this book. Please refer to the resources section of this book for information about these issues.

We often take our verbal abilities, and the ability to produce sounds easily and effortlessly, for granted. However, speech disorders call attention to themselves all the time. Spend any amount of time watching TV, and you will see an endless parade of children with lisps, /r/ distortions, immature sounding speech, and more. This is done on purpose by advertisers—it gets your attention. You can also look at news reporters to find another trove of issues, perhaps the most famous being Barbara Walters with her distortion of her /r/ sound. Tom Brokaw has a particular /l/ distortion that always makes me pay attention. It is for this reason that difficulties in this area should be addressed; how you pronounce your sounds should not detract from the message you are trying to convey.

While it is true that there is some variability in the age when children reach developmental milestones, we do have a general idea of when they should have particular sounds mastered. This can be used as a guidepost by you or your child's pediatrician or teacher to determine whether there is an issue that should be addressed. However, regardless of how many charts you consult, the main question you should ask yourself is, "Would someone less familiar with my child be able to understand what she is saying?" You can go further by asking yourself, "Does my child seem frustrated or shy about talking? Do people comment on her speech?" If you answered no to the first question and yes to the second, it may be time to take a closer look at this area.

As we discussed in the last chapter, a full and comprehensive evaluation will include a look at articulation, or how well your child is able to make sounds by themselves (that is, in *isolation*), or how well she is able to make these sounds in syllables, in words, and in sentences. The assessment process looks at all aspects of sound production from breath support to resonance (how nasal your speech sounds). We also look at the total number of sounds (vowels and consonants) in your child's repertoire and how she is able to use them in connected speech. We look for patterns of errors, as well as times when there is inconsistency. We examine the mouth and observe motor patterns during production of sounds, and we listen for a sense of overall clarity, or *intelligibility*, in conversation and context. This allows us to do a differential diagnosis of articulation difficulties; this is critical in determining the type, frequency, and content of the therapy program.

There are several different types of articulation disorder that we will discuss in this chapter, including: motor-based articulation disorders, phonological disorders, dysarthria (neurological and muscular), and apraxia. Let's look at each one in turn.

The first type of articulation disorder is a *motor-based articulation disorder*. This is a complex way of expressing that the primary problem is getting correct placement for making a particular sound, or moving the mouth in the correct way. The easiest and most common example of this is a lisp, where the child produces a /th/ sound instead of an /s/, saying "thmile" instead of "smile." This is a typical developmental error, but when it fails to self-correct, there is likely an underlying issue with the tongue or jaw that is maintaining an inappropriate and immature pattern. Another example would be a child who can produce all sounds except /r/, so that he sounds like Elmer Fudd, saying "that wascally wabbit." This is usually due to difficulty in shaping the back of the tongue to produce the /r/ sound, resulting in either the use of /w/ or more of an /eu/ sound, called a "retroflex" /r/. In some cases, children will have difficulty with producing a whole class of related sounds, such as /sh/, /ch/, and /j/, all sounds produced with specific tongue cupping, or all tongue tip sounds, like /l/, /s/, /t/, /d/, and /n/, produced by making contact between the tongue tip and the roof of the mouth.

For these children, it is important to determine where the glitch is in the speech-production system that is keeping them from getting motor control over the sound or sounds in error. We look at muscle tone, tongue-jaw differentiation, which movements are limited, and the pattern of errors. Does the child completely omit the sound? Or use a consistent substitute, as in the example of the lisp? Once we understand this, we can begin to teach the child correct placement, using muscle training and verbal and visual feedback to help him learn to make the sound. At the same time, we are teaching him to hear and see and feel how the sound is made correctly. Once he masters production of the sound in isolation, he practices producing the sound in increasingly complex contexts (such as phrases, sentences, or reading out loud) while learning to monitor his own productions. This practice should be intense as we are establishing a new motor program for the brain to run when that sound or sounds is required. Your SLP may ask you to help with homework or continued daily practice once a sound is coming along; the more frequent and intense the practice, the quicker the progress.

The second type of speech sound disorder is a *phonological disorder*. This can be thought of as more of a language-based issue, where children exhibit particular patterns of error that help to simplify speech production or show where they do not understand how sounds go together. These children can be very difficult to understand initially because there are usually multiple patterns operating simultaneously. Also, the errors shown by these children make speech easier to produce but harder to understand.

Evaluation for a phonological disorder is much the same as for an articulation disorder. You want to rule out any muscular involvement, and, typically, these kids can make their error sounds, but they don't use them appropriately in context. Examples of phonological errors include those of children who can't produce /k/ or /g/ and consistently use /t/ or /d/ instead, saying "tar" for "car," or those of children who are unable to produce any fricative/continuant sounds (such as f or sh) and always substitute a stop sound such as /p/, saying "pip" for "fish." See table 5.1 for examples of other patterns. The key to phonological disorders is their consistency and their predictability. They affect classes of sounds, not just a single sound and can have a significant impact on intelligibility.

Also see table 5.1 for some examples of the most common phonological processes.

Treatment for these children involves learning to hear the target sound or sounds, and then practicing the correct sound by contrasting it with the error sound. For example, a child who consistently uses /t/ and /d/ for /k/ and /g/ is using a process called *fronting*, where a sound that is supposed to be produced at the back of the mouth is made at the front of the mouth. In treatment, we would use a technique called *auditory bombardment*, where your child would have the opportunity to listen to many productions of their target sound, followed by structured practice using something we call "minimal pairs," or pairs of sounds that differ by only one feature, such as voicing.[1] This might involve playing a game where they would have to contrast use of words with the error sound and the target sound. An example would be having pictures of a *coat*

**Table 5.1.  Examples of Phonological Process Patterns**

| Process Name | Example | Description | When it typically disappears |
|---|---|---|---|
| Stopping | Dope for soap | Replacing a long or fricative sound with a short sound | Between 3 and 4 years |
| Final consonant deletion | Be/bed or ca/cat | Leaving off the final sound in a word | By age 3 |
| Fronting | Dat/cat or tape/cake | Replacing a back sound with one in the front | By age 3 |
| Gliding | Wemon/lemon or wabbit/rabbit | Replacing an l or r with a /w/ sound | 4 years |
| Assimilation | Tat/cat or pop/top | Making the 2 consonants in a word the same | By age 3 |
| Cluster reduction | Side/slide or bidge/ bridge | Eliminating l sound from a consonant cluster | By age 4.5 |

and a *tote*, and your child would have to correctly identify or produce one of the two. (Remember, these kids are capable of making the sound, they just don't use it correctly.) As treatment progresses, practice using the correct sound in more and more complex activities. In contrast to motor-based treatment, the work is with a class of sounds, rather than one sound at a time. This means that instead of working on how to elevate the tongue to say /l/, as in a motor-based disorder, he would practice /k/ and /g/ at the same time, contrasted with /t/ and /d/, the most common error pattern.

Some children also exhibit what we call "atypical phonological process" errors that are not usually seen in children as they develop their sound repertoire. These errors usually require more intensive treatment and may indicate a more complex disorder. At times, phonological disorders can co-occur with motor-based deficits, or apraxia.

A third type of speech disorder is *dysarthria*, which accompanies a neurological or muscle-based disorder. Dysarthria can affect all the systems of speech production, including breath support, resonance, voicing, and articulation.[2] While the main component of dysarthria is weakness (resulting in low volume and imprecise articulation), you may also see strain patterns or difficulty with coordinating systems for efficient speech production. Dysarthria is not a developmental condition, and it is typically seen in children with neuromuscular disorders such as cerebral palsy (CP), amyotrophic lateral sclerosis (ALS), spinal muscular atrophy (SMA), and the dystrophies.

Treatment for dysarthria usually involves looking at the systems that are involved, and determining which systems might respond to treatment aimed at strengthening or changing function, and which aspects require compensatory strategies or augmentative and alternative communication (AAC). For example, a child with poor breath support may be able to do some exercises that increase tidal volume (how much air is exchanged with each breath) and the amount of air used when speaking. In contrast, if his positioning impacts that child's breath support, using postural supports may allow him to better access what lung function he has. In further contrast, perhaps the low respiratory support stems from a medical condition that is not likely to change or improve. In that case, we would explore options, including technology (voice output systems) that could speak for him when he is unable to speak for himself.

In looking at dysarthria, we must carefully consider the impact of exercise and muscle training, since muscle fatigue and poor endurance can be significant obstacles. In many cases, we are working to teach a child how best to use the skills and capacity he has. It is important to work with other medical and therapeutic team members with these children, to ensure that we are getting the full picture and that we are providing for all their needs. It is also critical to remember that speech is only one way that we communicate; we use a variety of verbal and nonverbal strategies to express our wants, needs, ideas, and feelings. It would be unfair to put all the pressure on speech for this child, not taking into consideration the complexity of thoughts he may want to share. Using AAC and technology allows us to close the gap between what he is capable of expressing and what he may want to say.[3]

The fourth type of speech disorder that we are going to discuss is *apraxia*. Sometimes called "developmental apraxia," "verbal apraxia," or "dyspraxia," the commonly used term in 2016 is *childhood apraxia of speech* (CAS). This term is used to contrast this speech disorder with *acquired apraxia*, which can occur after a traumatic brain injury. CAS is a childhood speech disorder that involves the motor speech system and is primarily a problem of selecting and sequencing sounds in speech. The easiest way to think about apraxia is that it is like a disconnect between the motor strip in the brain and the mouth. A child may know what sounds she wants to make, but they come out garbled or in the wrong order. It is an issue of programming and sequencing sounds in speech, resulting in significant inconsistency and poor intelligibility.[4]

There is a significant spectrum of deficit with apraxia, from children who primarily have difficulty acquiring sounds to children who are unable to make sounds at all. In my clinical experience, it is also a disorder that evolves and changes over time and with treatment. Children who look very much like they fall into this category in their toddler years can look quite different by four years of age, particularly with good intervention. The hardest part of dealing with apraxia is that it can't necessarily be identified as a structural issue on a CT scan or an MRI, but it is thought to have a neurological basis. In addition, apraxia can be particularly challenging since children who are affected may have average to above average intelligence and normal receptive language skills, resulting in high levels of frustration.[5] However, it should also be noted that children who have many other disorders, including autism spectrum disorders, may *also* have apraxia, so careful diagnosis is key to getting the right treatment.

Children with apraxia can exhibit many different characteristics, beginning in infancy. As they grow and develop their language skills, there is often a gap between their understanding and what they can express. This causes them to limit how much they speak, or it impacts their ability to master aspects of language that allow them to progress to saying longer sentences. Another challenge seen with apraxia is its inconsistency. Not only do they exhibit different errors moment to moment and day by day, but they can sometimes produce a complex word or short sentence that they cannot do again when asked to do so. This is quite frustrating to many parents, as they express that "he said it over the weekend, why can't he say it again?"

The reason why he cannot say it again has to do with the nature of *spontaneous* versus *on demand* production. When a child is playing with words and sounds, he will often say something out of the blue, where there is no pressure and no particular forethought. However, when *asked* to produce something, he has to willingly activate his motor system; this is more complicated and for kids with apraxia, ripe with opportunities for breakdown. Imitation skills are hard to develop and maintain for this reason.[6]

Since imitation is a primary strategy in traditional articulation therapy ("watch me and do what I do"), we have to use different procedures and techniques to assist a child with apraxia to master sounds. In fact, we work on several goals at the same time, including:

- production of clear, differentiated vowels (since making correct vowel sounds contributes significantly to clarity);
- production of different syllable shapes (increasing the variety and complexity of how they can put sounds together);
- production of syllable rhythm;
- production of natural-sounding speech through pitch, intonation, syllable stress.

In the interest of being comprehensive, children with speech disorders can also include those who fail to develop sounds at all, but not due to any of the above issues. They may include children with permanent hearing loss, or those who have frequent ear infections, which result in fluctuating hearing loss. For these children, we work on awakening their awareness of their mouth and its sound-making abilities; this may include back-and-forth babbling, play with mouth toys and fingers, and playing vocal games. The goal of this process is to facilitate the normal progression of skills, from crying and production of neutral vowels (like an "uh" sound), to complex sequences of many different sounds.

Regardless of the type of speech sound disorder, there are some common aspects of treatment. First, all speech sound disorders require an element of education and teaching, whether to learn about the motor aspects of how the mouth needs to move or to learn to differentiate a correct sound from the error sound. In addition, all treatment programs typically require a *hierarchical approach*; that is, they progress from simple productions (sound or syllable in isolation) to more and more complex contexts. A child nearing the end of her program might focus on self-monitoring production of her target sound while reading out loud, while a child at the beginning of treatment might focus on production of her target consonant with different vowels.

In addition, programs used to treat speech sound disorders also require that the child learn to monitor her own productions so that she can self-correct when needed. This is important when sounds are generalized from structured tasks (including drill activities like naming pictures) to more functional communication (such as having a conversation with friends), where fewer prompts and supports are available. The ultimate goal is for your child to learn to use her new sound all the time, no matter what she is doing or trying to express. This is a big task, one that takes a lot of practice.

In my experience, speech sound disorders in children are often much more complex than the way these issues have been outlined here. In fact, many children exhibit aspects of one or more of these at the same time. This requires flexibility and good differential diagnosis by the SLP so that all aspects of speech production are addressed appropriately. There are many commercial programs available to SLPs to use with different types of speech disorders. For phonological disorders, the Hodson Cycles approach is well known[7]; there are also commercially available programs for lisp and /r/ distortion. For the child with multiple types of speech sound disorders, it is necessary that the SLP be able to incorporate elements of the various treatment approaches in ways that bring about the biggest functional change in intelligibility.

I would also like to note that it is important to ensure that your child's language is being addressed simultaneously with articulation issues or even before they are addressed. While there are some aspects of speech production that can be improved with very young children (such as pitch play, rhythmic sound production, and babbling), articulation therapy requires sustained attention and the language ability to make use of the instruction being provided. It is important that a child have something to say before we worry about how she says it; so be sure that language and communication is also being addressed. Again, the use of augmentative or alternative methods may be needed as a bridge while children are learning to speak. Given that the most important goal is that they be able to communicate their wants and needs, addressing language issues and providing a system of communication is critical.

If your child has been or is diagnosed with a speech sound disorder, here are some questions that you can ask your SLP, in order to get a better understanding of his or her difficulties:

1. What kind of speech sound disorder does my child have? Why do you think this is what is going on? What aspects of his speech led you to this diagnosis?
2. What sounds will my child work on? In what order?
3. What kind of program or approach are you using in treatment? Why?
4. What kind of supports and cues are you providing to help my child master new sounds?
5. What should I be doing at home? How much homework should I expect?
6. How would you describe my child's intelligibility? And what is the long-term goal for this program?
7. How will you teach me to carry over what you are doing in speech therapy?
8. How do I respond if my child makes his sound wrong during practice at home?

Addressing speech sound disorders in children helps them to acquire all the sounds for their primary language and allows them to communicate in a way that is consistent with their language level. Some children make rapid progress with intervention, while others may need years of treatment to reach completion. It is critical to partner with your SLP to help your child build his or her skills and feel successful. Although I said it before, it needs to be said again: For children working on speech sounds, there must be *daily practice* to make good progress. The more he works on it, the better it gets. The converse is also true: The less he practices, the longer it may take to reach mastery because he may be alternately practicing correct and incorrect patterns. In other words, the old pattern may still be getting reinforced. It is important to understand that no matter how skilled the SLP, articulation therapy without daily home practice is time and money wasted.

# 6

# AN OVERVIEW OF LANGUAGE DISORDERS

It is estimated that between six and eight *million* children in the Unites States have some form of language disorder.[1] This can range from a mild delay in getting started with language to a combination of language and other developmental problems to a medical or neurological condition that can significantly impede almost any development of language. This chapter will discuss each of these categories separately as their causes, treatments, and outcomes can be quite different. This chapter will also discuss the goals for treatment that might be targeted within various clinical settings. Having a solid understanding of how this process is driven from a clinical perspective will allow you to partner with your SLP for the benefit of your child.

The goal of any intervention for language disorders is to round out and equalize all the areas of language content, form, and use. Recall from earlier in the book that we discussed how language actually represents several categories of skills:

*Content*: The words we use, the meaning of our communication, and the ideas we express;

*Form*: How we construct our communication, the ways we communicate, and the complexity of what we can express; and

*Use*: The reasons we communicate and how successfully we navigate the social context of interaction.

This chapter will also provide a deeper look into the areas of language that are assessed and evaluated clinically, and how those results inform the goals that we select for treatment. Our primary goal is twofold: to establish missing foundation skills, and then to teach ways to compensate for skills that are not likely to develop or that may remain a relative weakness moving forward. We want to fill in the gaps, wherever possible, and provide ways to foster independence and success for those not filled. When children have language disorders, we must make explicit the things that are typically learned through observation and experience by children without such challenges. We must teach a child with a language disorder how to organize his world, and put words to his experiences, so that he can express himself in meaningful ways.

## DEVELOPMENTAL DELAY—THE LATE TALKER

For some children, learning to express themselves does not come easily. Although we often do not know the reason for this delay, they fail to develop vocabulary and seem frustrated in their attempts to communicate with others. Some children in this situation have strong receptive language skills, while others have equal weakness in their receptive and expressive skills. We can discuss each in turn.

A child who has strong receptive language skills seems to understand everything that is said to him. He is able to identify body parts and familiar people, and he can often do things on command (as long as it is not saying a word); he seems very bright. Such children often use elaborate means, including pantomime, guiding you to what he wants, or using gestures to let you know what he wants or needs. In addition, he may also be very skilled at getting others, such as siblings or a caring parent, to be his voice. Because he is so bright, it can be easy to overlook his difficulties for quite some time. He may manage to get by quite well until his second year, when he begins to seek more independence and wants to assert his own agenda. It is often at this point, when frustration begins to occur more frequently, that you may identify a problem and seek help. Your initial conversations with a spouse or physician may yield a recommendation to wait it out and see how he progresses over the next six months or more. I highly recommend that you seek help, even for a young child. Why wait and let the problem get worse?

Intervention for children with an isolated expressive language delay is fairly straightforward. Our primary goal is to activate the child's inner drive to use words and sentences to achieve what she has been doing through nonverbal means. In my work with parents and families, this involves training the parent as much as the child. In the earliest stages of intervention, this typically means helping parents and children tune in to one another. Often, children are using signals and attempting to communicate, but because it does not sound like words, or look like communication, signals can get missed. I help parents tune in to their child, and learn to observe and interpret the ways in which she is already communicating. Then we can begin to establish more conventional, recognizable words and gestures. Next, we move to structure the environment, at home and in therapy, to foster as many opportunities for communication as possible. We want to create reasons for your child to communicate and to set her up for success. We also gradually change the expectations, so that successful communication happens only when verbal attempts are made. Finally, we work on activities that build vocabulary and provide a highly motivating context for words to emerge. Once words have emerged and are being used in simple combinations, we can use techniques such as *expansion*, and *expansion plus correction*, to enhance the complexity of what they are able to say. Finally, we work on supporting the use of words in various social contexts and with varying levels of demands.[2]

When I speak with parents about a child at this stage, I often speak about the process of helping her discover her power as a communicator. For any child, she first learns that communication helps her to regulate the behavior of others. The thinking process might be, "Hmmmm. When I do this, things happen. My favorite person or toy appears." It is a special honor to see how children make this discovery and begin to emerge into the world in a very different way. In fact, once a child begins to use her verbal skills more confidently, I usually hear parents ask, "Where is the off switch? Now that she is talking, she never stops!"

Helping children acquire words and the social savvy to use them can involve several different stages or techniques. One of the ones I use most often in my practice is sign language. For a child who has strong receptive language skills and knows what she wants to say but lacks the ability to produce words consistently, sign language provides a critical bridge to success and independence. Many parents question whether using signs will discourage the development of speech because it gives her a way out of trying to use words. Fortunately, both the research and my own clinical experience prove the opposite is actually true.[3]

Allowing and encouraging the use of sign language serves as a bridge, not a crutch. I have seen countless children take to sign language so quickly that they begin "saying" words no one even knew they knew. The frustration that had been so prominent begins to decrease, and everyone in that child's life now has another means of connecting. What usually happens is that the sign allows her to get what she wants or needs but removes the pressure of trying to say words. However, she is also hearing the words with the signs, and a deeper connection is made between sign and word. Over time, the word and sign will likely be produced together, and then the sign drops away when the word is mastered. I have seen this happen even with children who have hearing loss and may need sign language as a support for a longer period of time. For children with normal hearing, and whose verbal skills are emerging, there is nothing more efficient than saying a word. Even though the use of sign language has become very popular, for children with and without delays, there are still likely to be many people in the child's life who do not know sign language. Children are driven to have their needs met, and they want to do that with minimal effort and stress.

One caveat about introducing signs, which I highly recommend: Be sure that whichever program or book you choose to use is based on American Sign Language (ASL) and not one of the very popular "baby sign" programs. These programs and resources for parents use iconic and simplified signs that resemble ASL, but sometimes unknowingly teach something that is actually an ASL sign for something you would not choose to teach your child. This can lead to confusion and embarrassment if you or your child use these signs in public and accidentally offend someone who uses ASL as a primary language. A few years ago, a parent I began working with told me that she had bought a book to try some baby signs with her daughter while she was waiting to be assigned an SLP. She was in a fast-food restaurant with her daughter, and she signed to see if her daughter wanted a "drink." She did not realize that there was another parent in line who was deaf, with her child. When she asked her daughter if she wanted a drink using the made up "baby sign," she was stunned be confronted by this other parent, and then to learn that this particular "baby sign" was actually an ASL sign for a graphic sex act! See the resources section toward the back of this book for some parent-tested, SLP-approved sign language resources.

Another stage in this process of working with late talkers is helping to shape the expectations about what counts as a word, and what to accept as a word when encouraging the child to be more verbal. From a language development perspective, when a child consistently uses a sound or combination of sounds to represent something, that counts as a word. This is true even if the sounds are incorrect at the early stage. Some examples would be if a child says "woof woof" for dog. Whenever they see a dog or someone mentions a dog, this is what you hear. Another example would be a child who says "Boppa" for his grandfather, when it is supposed to be "Papa." We give credit for the consistency and forgive the form or sound errors, given his rapidly developing sound system. Another example would be all the ways that children begin to label me, Suzanne Ducharme, the speech pathologist. I have been every version of "Sue," which is what I usually have children call me. I have been called Shoe, Pooh, Too, Boo, Do, Zoo. . . . These errors demonstrate the ways that articulation can impact language. However, a child may use this sound combination to greet me, to label me, and even to request me. It clearly becomes his way of identifying who I am for himself and others.

In contrast, a combination of sounds would not count as a word if it were used universally. This would be the case if a child used a generic "buh" or "dat" to refer everything. Parents are sometimes able to discern what a child talking about by using context (what he is looking at, pointing to) or tone of voice. Some children manage to insert "fifty shades" of meaning into a single syllable, but this would not count as a word from a clinical perspective. We would work to shape that single syllable into different words and to expand vocabulary to promote communication effectiveness by making meaning more clear.

Understanding this process of how sounds become words, and what counts as a word, makes it easier to understand how you might respond to your child's attempts as he moves through the process of treatment. What I try to emphasize with parents is to *validate the content and model the form*. When he has used a clear word for something, even if the sounds are not perfect, let him know you understand what he is trying to say while modeling the correct way to say it. The exchange might go something like this:

Child: "Ootie." While signing or pointing to a cookie.

Adult: Oh! You want a cookie! C-ookie."

Child: "C-ookie" while reaching for the cookie.

Once a child begins to develop a core vocabulary, and he experiences success at using words and making things happen, he will, hopefully, begin to attempt to say more words, more frequently. Activities to increase imitation are also very useful at this stage because a child can, hopefully, use imitation as a learning strategy to further expand his vocabulary. There is usually a tipping point where it seems as if there is a cascade of new words that emerge very quickly. This is often the *lexical burst* that was discussed earlier in the book; this signals a readiness for the next stage of language, which is *word combinations*.

In my experience, the mastery of single words can be a slow process at first. Likewise, the step up from single words to two-word combinations can also seem quite effortful. Our efforts in treatment focus on modeling two-word utterances and showing how to combine words to achieve new goals. In many instances, however, moving from two words to three words and beyond seems to happen much more easily and quickly.

When working to move children to two-word combinations, we are able to use many consistent anchor words to generate these combinations. This means that we combine words in predictable ways, using certain words that combine easily with many other words. In our training as SLPs, we learn about Brown's Semantic Relations, which outlines *some* of these early combinations as follows:[4]

Agent-action: Car go! Ball roll! Dada eat.
Action-object: Go car! Eat cookie?
Agent-object: Mama car!
Entity-locative: Ball table (The ball is on the table) or Dada work?
   (Dad is at work?)
Possesser-possession: My sock. Dada car.

I have found it helpful to teach parents the following connector words to make many two-word combinations:

More _____All done _____
   Where _____? My/your _____
   Color/shape _____ please.
   Size _____Go _____
   _____ go!Hi/Bye _____
   No _____ _____ all gone.

We also want to target typical phrases such as "My turn," "I want," and others. Simultaneously, we are working on consistent use of "yes" and "no" and providing as many verbal means as possible for the child to communicate his wants and needs.

Once children begin to combine words more consistently, *grammar* emerges. We begin to see pluralization (the use of —s) and the use of —ing at the end of words to show action (walking). This is also a time when your child may begin to use more than two words to request or label things she sees. There is a predictable progression of how grammatical structures emerge, and your SLP can guide you in observing and facilitating the development of these forms. By the age of three years, most children are already marking plural (/s/, /z/, /es/) and actions with —ing, as well as early pronouns (I, you, me, my, mine) and possession (Emma's turn).

For children who have weaknesses in both understanding and expressive skills, the strategies and goals are largely the same, with the addition of specific work to build their listening skills and, over time, improve the ability to process information of increasing length and increasing complexity. For such children, focusing and sustaining attention can be quite challenging. In my clinical experience, we often have to determine whether the "attention issue" is due to typical developmental focus on motor skills, or represents a true deficit in selecting and staying with one thing at a time. For those children who truly struggle with attention in the toddler years, part of an SLP's work is to help a child develop listening skills and learn to attach meaning to what she hears.

When I first began practicing in 1994, no child with a suspected speech and language delay was seen for an evaluation without having a *full* hearing test with an audiologist. This allowed us to know, from the beginning, that hearing loss was not a contributing factor in the speech or language delay. Today, in 2016, this is no longer the gold standard, and many parents are told that if their child passed the newborn hearing screening, then hearing is most likely fine. The fact is that some types of hearing loss occur after the newborn period, and many children suffer from ear infections and other ear problems that *can* affect their speech and language development. If your child has difficulty with understanding language or focusing her attention or seems to have trouble hearing, continue to advocate strongly with your pediatrician that a hearing test *must* be conducted. (If you go to a speech and language evaluation and have not had one, the SLP is likely to recommend that you have one, just to be sure.)

Although a comprehensive discussion of hearing loss is beyond the scope of this book, it is important to mention that being able to detect loud sounds, or even softer sounds, in the environment ("He can hear me when I bang pots." or "He is bothered by sirens.") is *not the same* as being able to hear and process speech sounds. Even the child who can hear a bag of potato chips being opened a room away may still have hearing difficulties that can affect his ability to learn speech and language. This is because most speech sounds are in the higher frequencies, meaning that they are very high pitched and very soft. A middle ear infection, or even frequent bouts of uninfected fluid, can block the child's ability to hear and perceive these important, softer speech sounds. Over time, a child who has chronic fluid can have moderate to severe issues with understanding what is said.[5] For those of you who watched *Peanuts* in the 1970s, think of how the teacher (or any adult) sounded to the kids. This will give you an idea of what ear fluid can do to your ability to understand speech. You know someone is talking, but it is impossible to make out the individual words and sounds to be able to respond appropriately.

Work on the development of listening and understanding skills might involve several areas, including building vocabulary (being able to identify people, objects, descriptors), following directions of increasing length and increasing complexity, developing an understanding of concepts (spatial, descriptive, quantity), and learning how to be a good conversation partner by responding appropriately. SLPs use a variety of techniques to build these skills and to practice them in both structured and unstructured tasks. For example, if your child is working on following single-step directions, you might practice this in Simon Says (highly structured activity), in an art activity (semi-structured) or in gross-motor play (unstructured.) Be sure to ask your SLP which listening/receptive skills are being addressed and how to support practice of these skills at home.

If your child has a medical or developmental reason why these skills may develop more slowly, or require more support, your child may also be taught compensatory strategies to help her manage spoken language. This may include things such as *reauditorization/rehearsal* (repeating a direction or piece of information to help remember it), *chunking* (putting pieces of information together to make fewer bits), or *visualization* (keeping a mental picture of what needs to be remembered). Your SLP may also teach you ways to give information or directions to your child that are designed to support her in this weaker area.

## NON-DEVELOPMENTAL LANGUAGE DISORDERS

Many late talkers have no known medical or neurological reasons for their delays, and they typically move through the normal stages of development, but at a slower pace or at a later time. The second group of children with language disorders includes those who have a medical, developmental, or neurological condition that also impacts the development of speech and language skills. Examples of this include *selective language impairment* and *developmental delay*, when all systems of development may be impacted. In some cases, we may know the cause of the language disorder, but in other situations, we never know the underlying cause of the disruption across systems.

In contrast to the late talkers, these children do not just move through the typical stages of development more slowly or at a later time. They struggle to develop skills and especially to access and apply them in social and learning situations. It is more common for them to have difficulties with *both* understanding and expression and to have other difficulties, such as attention deficits and sensory processing issues, that impact the ability to tune into and make use of language in the activities of everyday life. For these kids, the struggle can show up in all areas, including content, form, and use, and it usually does.

Take Jake, a little boy I started seeing when he was three years old. He had been in early intervention but had made minimal progress. Jake had a few words, and he could combine some of them. He could follow simple directions, like "stop" and "come here," but struggled with longer directions. He did not learn new things easily, and his speech was hard to understand. Jake also had low muscle tone, which made movement difficult, and sensory processing issues that made him sensitive to most things in the environment. He was easily frustrated, and it took him many repetitions to learn something, and even more to retain it. In short, most everything seemed to be a struggle for this little boy.

Our work together focused on the basics, initially. We worked on learning vocabulary so that he could label and ask for things. We worked on attention and completing activities. We used visuals and sign language to reduce his frustration, and we helped him learn to follow directions. Later, we worked in improving his oral motor skills (nasal breathing, better airflow for speech, specific lip and tongue movements needed to make sounds) and his articulation to help him speak more clearly.

Once he had mastered the basic skills, we worked on later developing language skills to help him produce sentences, to engage in conversation, and to process longer and more complex directions and information. We helped him to develop his auditory-based pre-reading skills and to begin to use his spoken language to direct his early efforts with written language. We also worked on understanding the structure of narratives and how to produce them. Jake was able to build many skills and use them successfully, but he also required compensatory strategies as well.

Through all of his hard work on his speech and language skills, we also had to work to compensate for his sensory-processing, attention, and movement challenges. For Jake, learning was not simply exposure and practice; we had to make accommodations for his learning style and to teach him the skills involved with how to learn. He struggled with frustration and therapy fatigue, and he often wished out loud that he did not have to come for speech anymore. Helping to support his self-esteem and his ability to persevere was as much a part of his therapy as any vocabulary activity.

In looking at the example of Jake, it is easy to see how the goals we discussed with regard to late talkers can be expanded and magnified for children with more complex issues. While we still want to establish those foundation skills, such as vocabulary, following directions, developing grammar for more complex sentences, and social use of language, we do so within a more challenging context. Sensory and medical issues sometimes result in changes to the sequence in which skills are introduced, or the way in which we teach or reinforce skills. In addition, SLPs (and you as parent) will likely need to provide more emotional supports, including counseling or modeling to help your child succeed.

In children with this level of deficit, you are much more likely to be working with a team of professionals, including physical and occupational therapists. Each professional will work on a different aspect of your child's development, and you will be providing support across the board. It may be helpful to work with your SLP to look at your *whole* child and to see how language and communication issues impact every aspect of his development. Your SLP may need to provide strategies to the other therapists about the most successful ways to provide directions to your child, or how to help him recall information to complete tasks. It will be critical for all therapists working with your child to understand how his speech and language skills are impacting his participation in all therapies, and how best to support him, regardless of the task he faces.

Jade, a little girl of twenty-two months, provides another example. She has had some medical challenges, and she has significant sensory issues, in that she is very sensitive to sounds, smells, and many types of touch. Her expressive language has been emerging, and she has some words, but she often uses them in ways that do not make sense. For example, when she is feeling stressed, she starts to sing "Let It Go" from the movie *Frozen*. She often does not respond to directions and sometimes not even to her name. She often seems overwhelmed, and her parents have to work hard at keeping her from having a meltdown. Her experiences with other therapists have often been unsuccessful and stressful for both Jade and her parents. This is partly because all of her services are delivered *via language*. None of these skilled and well-meaning therapists were taking into consideration how hard it is for Jade to process language and for her to access her language skills to respond appropriately. Once she gets overwhelmed, it is hard to bring her back due to her sensory issues and difficulty in organizing herself. By shifting *how* they speak to her and *how* they try to engage with her,

her therapists can experience much more success in helping her build and practice the skills she needs to learn.

The main focus for children with speech and language impairments embedded in a more complex developmental picture is on developing functional communication. As they develop more skills, the focus shifts to increasing the complexity of their language and the social context where they can successfully use it. Finally, SLPs also focus on laying the foundation needed for mastery of pre-academic skills in the preschool child, and those needed to access and master curricular content in the grade school, middle school, or high school child. This can mean a shift from verbal language to reading and written language, since the demands for these more advanced skills increase as children progress in school.

School-based SLPs focus on many aspects of speech and language development, depending on the type of school and the size of their caseload. While some members of the public may mistakenly believe that SLPs in the schools are only used to "fix lisps and problems with /r/," they perform a vital function in the school by acting as a liaison between a language-disordered child and his teachers and other therapists. The school SLP plays a critical role in helping children learn content-based vocabulary and learn and apply compensatory strategies in the classroom and in teaching the teachers how to support that language disordered child in all aspects of his school experiences. The goals set by the team each year reflect the need to help each child access the curriculum and interact with peers within the school environment.

SLPs who are in private practice can, and often do, support children who also receive services in school. If the speech and language services are paid for by your insurance carrier, the SLP will help with disorders that also meet the definition of "medical necessity" and impact your child's processing or expressive abilities. If you pay privately, you will have more leeway with determining the kinds of goals you address. As a private practitioner, I can address academic and medical issues equally, and use more creativity in how I teach skills, because I only have to answer to the parent.

In either setting, the SLP will work with you and your child to help build skills that are missing, to develop increasingly sophisticated communication skills, and to develop reasoning and problem-solving skills that are used across all the aspects of everyday life. SLPs also provide emotional support and guidance for the development of your child's self-esteem, and help address any issues with bullying that may come up.[6]

## SEVERE LANGUAGE IMPAIRMENT

For children who are born with serious medical or neurological conditions, such as cerebral palsy, Down syndrome, or stroke, developing language is often seen as more of a long-term goal. The focus for these children is usually on getting medically stable first, and then developing some core skills such as head control, feeding skills, or walking. Communication is sometimes disregarded or minimized as an option, given all of the medical concerns to be addressed. In my clinical opinion, this is unfair and shortsighted.

For these children, developing language and communication skills is more effortful and time-consuming than for either of the previous types of language disorders we have discussed. This is because a child's neurological and medical status makes him less available for the early bonding experiences that lead to the development of these skills. In addition, his ongoing difficulties with motor development can make it difficult to teach him signs or gestures and for him to master even things like facial expressions. Frankly, I often find that there is an expectation that language or communication is not likely, so it is left out of the vision. Many of these children can spend months or years, being moved through their lives, where everything is treated as a medical procedure, from G-tube feeds to dressing, and there is limited opportunity to develop communication skills.

It is true that such a child would tend to use crying as a primary means of communicating because it is what he has available to him. All babies start this way. But give even the newest mom a few weeks, and she can tell all the nuances of her baby's cry. The same can usually be said for children with severe impairments, but the subtle signals will be missed unless you know what to look for and how to respond. A good SLP can help you tune in to all the signals your baby is giving you and help you develop those early cycles of engagement that lead to communication. Perhaps your baby likes a particular kind of touch, and you can use that to help them vocalize for more. Another example would be figuring out the kinds of stimulation that trigger a meltdown in your baby and knowing how to avoid them to keep him calm and allow him to sleep for longer periods.

The bottom line for severely impaired children is that you need someone to help you tune in to your baby and to develop a communication system that allows him to interact with his world, even in small ways. Over time, your SLP can work with you to develop a total communication system that may include what we call Augmentative and Alternative Communication (AAC). There is a whole subset of SLP professionals who do this kind of work exclusively, focused on choosing, and teaching you and your child how to use, various types of technology for communication. Some children use voice output devices, or apps that provide spoken language while he develops his speech skills, while other children may need these devices for a lifetime.

However, even if your child needs and uses an AAC device, he will need to master all the same prerequisite behaviors as children with more typical language development and to have reasons to communicate. These children also need to learn vocabulary, master concepts, and learn how to interact. However, at the same time, they must also learn how to use their technology purposefully. SLPs are critical members of the team for children with severe medical and neurological conditions from the very beginning. They are there to support you in tuning in to your child, in developing a mutual communication system and in supporting your child's development as he grows up.

## SPECIAL POPULATIONS: AUTISM SPECTRUM DISORDERS

Autism spectrum disorders (ASD) represents one of the fastest growing diagnostic groups in the world today. According to the Autism Society of America, one in sixty-eight children in the United States is diagnosed with autism, representing over 3.5 million people.[7] Recent changes in the way autism is diagnosed are still being worked out, but in my experience, there is no diagnosis that strikes more fear and anguish in a parent's heart than autism.

Our understanding of what autism is, what might be causing it, and how we treat it is rapidly evolving. It was initially thought that withdrawn mothers (called "refrigerator mothers") might cause autism,[8] but now it is understood as a brain-based disorder that likely has a genetic component. In fact, there is research looking into many potential causes, including an excess of unused brain cells or the triggering of genetically compromised systems by environmental toxins.[9]

Regardless of the reason for autism, we know that it is a spectrum of disorders, thus the abbreviation ASD, with some common core features. These include, but are not limited to:

- persistent deficits in social communication and interaction;
- restricted, repetitive patterns of behavior, interests, or activities;
- difficulty with language development and play skills;
- an onset in early childhood.

A diagnosis of autism also now includes a designation of severity, based on the level of support a child will need to achieve some level of functional ability.[10]

From an SLP perspective, our role with children who have autism spectrum disorder is not all that different from our role with children with other types of language disorders. In practical ways, however, our methods and our strategies may look different. This is because of the understanding we now have about how children with ASD learn and how they must work to generalize that learning across contexts. SLPs can help with the development of verbal and nonverbal skills, help parents tune in to what their children are trying to communicate, and help with the development of foundation skills that help children to develop a language system. SLPs also have a role in the development of play skills (the seed from which language grows) and social skills (learning how to interact with others) and with how the children can manage their own emotions and stay regulated and available for learning.

One of my struggles as an SLP has been with the proliferation of the use of applied behavioral analysis (ABA) for children with autism. Conventional wisdom has held for some time, particularly in ABA circles, that ABA is the only effective tool for children with autism and that high-intensity treatment, sometimes in excess of thirty hours per week, is necessary.[11] For a developing and already compromised brain, that feels like a level of intensity that might actually work against development. As you recall, stressed systems don't strengthen. This is not to say that many children have not benefited from ABA services, or that ABA is not an important part of the team. However, in some cases, ABA staff may unknowingly influence a parent to believe that ABA alone will result in progress and that ABA is sufficient to develop speech and language skills. And due to the intense time commitment for ABA, some parents actually stop their SLP services.

ABA master therapists are trained in learning theory and in the principles of ABA. Their primary function is to teach a child the foundation skills he needs to be available for learning and to master basic skills. The master therapist oversees a team of ABA interventionists, who may have only a high school education. These providers are taught to carry out behavior programs and are supervised by the master therapist and may not have had any training in working with children or in child development. This is also true for the knowledge of communication development and disorders.

Remember that SLPs are, at a minimum, master's level–trained clinicians with specific emphasis on the development of speech and language, with broad skills in managing deficits regardless of the diagnosis. Not only is there room for both at the table, there is *need* for both at the table. If your child is diagnosed with autism, make sure you have ample opportunity to work with an SLP; we are the professionals with specific training in this area who can help guide you through that aspect of your child's development.

In my experience, working with children with ASD involves both specific intervention for language development and a special focus on the development of social skills. Children with ASD may also require assistance with the development of speech, and many have apraxia (see chapter 5 for more information). Some children will require AAC devices or technology as part of their overall communication system. Regardless of the specific difficulties in question, SLPs always strive to build what skills we can, teach compensatory strategies to overcome the gaps, teach parents and others how to facilitate language and set up the environment to support communication, and offer support around self-regulation and organization.

## SPECIAL POPULATIONS: PREMATURE INFANTS

Over 15 million infants are born prematurely each year, according to the March of Dimes.[12] Any baby born at less than thirty-seven weeks gestation is considered preterm, although some babies are now surviving birth at twenty-four or twenty-five weeks gestation. Having worked with many babies in the neonatal intensive care unit (NICU), and later in my practice with them as toddlers, I feel it is important to include some discussion of them in this chapter. This is because, despite the fact that many of these babies do well long term, they still carry what I call the "preemie legacy" that impacts their neurological organization and, thus, their language skills for years after the medical complications are conquered.

Premature birth affects many aspects of a child's development, but it all starts with the brain. As you may recall from chapter 2, we are born with billions of brain cells that grow, change, and connect during the first few years of life. For premature infants, this process is interrupted by an early birth, and the brain is subject to multiple, ongoing, and often unpleasant stimuli. This might include surgery, invasive testing procedures, and even being in the NICU itself. What results is a brain that is dominated by stress-mediated pathways, while the parts of the brain that control relaxation and emotional control are less active than they would be in a full-term baby.[13]

This tendency to upset easily, to be more stressed overall, and to have more difficulty in regulating after an upset can last for years. From a speech and language perspective, it can affect several areas, including:

- Parent-infant bonding: Premature babies do not behave like full-term babies do, and often in the midst of the crisis, parents are not taught about the special ways they need to interact with their baby. When they inevitably do what parents do with a newborn baby, they are greeted with withdrawal, stress, or even episodes where the baby stops breathing or her heart rate drops. This mismatch impacts the bonding process because parents can sometimes feel discouraged or rejected. Thus, the initial development of cycles of engagement that lead to mutual vocal play and proto-conversations later are interrupted.

- Medical fragility and even nutritional or feeding issues make babies less available for developmental work, due to weakness, illness, or frequent hospitalization. This often means long periods with limited contact or altered mobility. Exploring the world through taste, touch, and movement is the basis for play skills, which in turn drive language development.
- Parental response to the fact and experience of premature birth: Many parents who have been through this experience have medical complications of their own, or have feelings that go unresolved from those early days. What stays prominent is the fear that something bad will happen, or that the baby will get sick or die. These understandable, but complicating, fears lead to differences in how parents interact with their children, sometimes resulting in permissive but restrictive practices. This can mean anything from limiting interactions (due to germ exposure) to limiting movement, and thus play, due to concerns about safety.
- Overall differences in sensory processing and regulation make some children less available for speech and language learning, or to experiences in general. For children who are hypersensitive to noise, light, touch, or movement, parenting becomes a minefield of potential triggers that can cause a meltdown or withdrawal completely. This in turn impacts how play skills develop, how a child interacts socially, and how he is able to participate in a variety of typical kid experiences like arts and crafts, going to the beach, or learning to ride a bike or play on a slide.

As SLPs, one of our primary roles is to assist kids to be comfortable with different kinds of sensory input and assist parents with how to regulate the level of arousal through modifying the home or therapy setting to avoid triggers. We also help parents understand the child's behavior and interpret his communication, verbal and nonverbal, during challenging experiences. We work to develop skills as close to the developmental guidelines as possible, while mitigating any factors that might interfere with learning. We also work closely with other professionals to develop the whole child and maximize their ability to participate in home, school, and community life. All of the other roles described above also apply to preemies as well.

## EVALUATION OF LANGUAGE DISORDERS

As discussed in chapter 4, speech and language evaluations vary from child to child and from professional to professional. The goal of any evaluation is to determine what functional skills are in place, what skills are missing, and what supports are needed to achieve the best functional outcome. We use the developmental framework and consider the mastery of milestones as a guide to know where a child *is* relative to where he should be. We also consider the impact of any medical, neurological, or other conditions on the child's status and prognosis. To briefly recap, SLPs may look at any or all of the following areas when they do an evaluation:

- receptive language: what words your child understands, how he follows directions, what concepts he knows, his processing speed and accuracy, his memory skills, and his comprehension of stories and questions;
- expressive language: words your child uses (vocabulary), syntax (how he uses grammar), his sentence types and structures, his social communication skills, his ability to generate stories, his skills in answering and asking questions, his functions of communication (why he communicates), and his reasoning and problem-solving skills;
- executive functioning skills: how your child approaches tasks, and organizes himself in time and space; his problem-solving skills and his ability to manage his behavior and predict the consequences of his actions.

Testing that takes place in a speech and language evaluation can include formal standardized tests, informal tests (checklists and special tasks), and clinical observations and parent reports. All of the information is taken together and used to develop a picture of your child's strengths and weaknesses as well as your child's learning style and task approach. Once this is complete, the SLP can determine an overall speech and language diagnosis, including information about severity and contributing factors. By considering the complete picture, SLPs can then develop a plan for intervention that considers what kind of strategies will best support your child in learning new skills, how to help him or her generalize those skills, and how to teach you to support his or her learning as well.

Recalling that our primary purposes are to develop skills where possible, and compensate for the rest, we see how a plan can begin to take shape. Typically, children work on many goals at the same time, so communication with your SLP is important. In my practice, I generally work with receptive language skills and understanding first, and then move to expression of the word, concept, or idea. For older children, I try to incorporate aspects of both into any activity, so that there is as much opportunity to work with the target goal as possible. For example, if we are working on mastery of spatial concepts, including words such as *in, on, under* and *behind*, we might start with a game I call "backward hide and seek." This means that rather than hiding objects around the room for him to find, I will tell the child where to put the items. This requires him to process both the location and the spatial word. ("Put the cup *under the chair.*") Later, to give him practice with labeling spatial words, I might ask him to recall where each item was, or I might allow him to "be the teacher" and tell me where to put the objects.

If your child has a language disorder, here are some questions you can ask your SLP:

- Does my child have a problem with receptive language, expressive language, or both?
- How would you describe my child?
- What skills does my child have? Where is he doing well? What are his relative strengths?
- What are the weakest areas?
- How do these areas or skills impact his overall competence as a communicator?
- What goals will you be addressing to start?
- Why are you choosing these goals? How will these goals support his development?
- What kind of strategies and cues will you use?
- What can I do to support him at home?

This chapter has provided an overview of language disorders, including some of the primary types: late talkers, children with communication problems embedded in a larger disorder, and severely impaired children with medical and neurological diagnoses. There was also a discussion of children with ASD and the lingering issues for children born prematurely. SLPs use a variety of diagnostic tools to determine a child's language profile, including relative strengths and weaknesses, as well as medical, sensory, or neurological factors that may be contributing to the difficulties. An intervention plan is developed based on an understanding of the complete profile, aimed at developing skills and teaching compensatory strategies to allow your child to develop the most functional skills possible. It is important to work with your SLP to determine the best way to support your child's language development and enhance his or her overall communication skills in an ongoing process as your child grows and evolves.

# Part II

# 7

# THE PARENT EXPERIENCE

**N**ow that you have identified a problem, and perhaps received a speech and language diagnosis, you can expect a whole new set of questions and challenges to arise. This chapter and the ones that follow are written specifically for you—to provide you with some information and guidance about how the experience of having a child with an identified special need may impact you in all the roles you serve, from parent to spouse to daughter or son. It is my hope that these chapters will be a source of comfort because I have seen firsthand how helpful it is to have a deep sense that you are understood and accepted as you are.

I am not a marriage and family counselor, nor am I a psychologist. However, counseling parents around issues that are related to a child's communication disorder *is* within my scope of practice. In fact, it represents a significant portion of what I do with families, and it is one of the primary reasons I wanted to write this book. And because so many issues arise when there is a child with communication issues, families over the years have taught me how important it is to directly address emotional and informational needs in addition to the clinical ones. In the process, I have learned a lot about how families function and what kinds of qualities seem to dominate in those that look and feel the most "successful," as defined by their own measures of happiness and perspective. It is these skills and traits that I wish to share with you. In addition, as a certified Holistic Manifestation Method Coach™, I am able to help parents clarify their vision, heal limiting beliefs, and release pain and take steps to manifest their vision.

However, when I feel like more specific help is needed, I can always refer to my colleagues in the counseling world to further support parents.

The first and most important thing that I can tell you is that you are going to be okay. Whatever you are feeling is acceptable and worthy of being heard and validated. Millions of others have been in your place, and they have felt everything you are feeling, from despair and anger to hope. Accept what you feel. Name it. Find ways to express your feelings to those who can be a source of support for you, and know that your feelings will not always be what they are now. Your feelings about yourself, your spouse, and your child will evolve in layers, impacted by your history and your personality. You will change, too, as will your spouse, your other children, and your extended family from the fact that you have a child with communication and developmental challenges. This process may not always be easy, but it can be positive and offer opportunities you may have missed given different circumstances.

## DEALING WITH THE DIAGNOSIS

Many parents describe similar responses to getting an "official diagnosis" for their child. It begins with the nagging fear or concern that something is wrong, which can often be met with resistance from family members and even pediatricians. That fear, or instinct, can lead to sleeplessness, marital conflict, and stress. Once the decision to have an evaluation or participate in medical testing is made, that fear can sometimes intensify with the looming unknown. This can also be exaggerated if there is another child within the family who has issues, or if there is a strong family history of a particular diagnosis, such as dyslexia or autism.

The path to completing all the necessary steps to arriving at a diagnosis can also be long and circuitous. In some cases, a visit to an SLP is all it takes to identify the problem and start moving toward a plan of intervention. In other cases, it may take visits to several different professionals and extensive medical testing to arrive at a unifying diagnosis. Frequently, there is a time lag between appointments and waiting for results that can be quite frustrating. During this process, all the emotions that led you to seek help are still present and may be intensified;

there may be little time to address them while you are busy managing the logistics of care for your child without supports.

Many parents describe the meeting where they received a diagnosis in a similar way: as if they wandered into a tunnel where time slows down, and it is hard to hear what the professionals are saying. It is a white-hot rush of adrenalin, and processing information is nearly impossible. Many emotions also come up at this time, such as:

- *Relief*: I was right. Something is wrong with my child.
- *Pain*: Oh no. Something is wrong with my child.
- *Fear*: What happens now? What does this mean? Will she ever . . . ?
- *Anger*: Why me? Why is this happening to my child?
- *Guilt*: Did I do something to cause this? Were my genes responsible for this? My spouse's?
- *Overwhelm*: How will I handle this? What will I need to do?
- *Grief*: This was not part of the plan. This was not supposed to happen.

There may be many more emotions, but this captures the essence of what I often hear. Know that it is perfectly all right that you need some time to process how you are feeling and this new information before you move forward. I recommend that you give yourself time to feel all that you are feeling, then find support and *then* get organized. There will be plenty of time for logistics when you are ready. As you move through this process, you will feel many different emotions, many in conflict with each other. Realize that this is perfectly normal. It is also normal to re-experience a feeling you thought you had already resolved. In my experience, these things come in waves, and there is no straight line. Being gentle with yourself, and reaching out for help as needed will keep you from getting stuck along the way.

**Experience:** Take a moment to close your eyes. Take a deep breath. Ask yourself, what emotion is asking to be expressed in this moment? Allow whatever comes up to be recognized. Name the emotion. Is it fear, anger, hope? Now ride that emotion. Don't try to stop it or judge it. Ride the wave of that emotion as it crests. It takes just ninety seconds for an emotion to reach a peak and then dissipate, and allowing the feeling to be expressed is healthy and critical to your mental and physical health.[1] (See appendix B for a worksheet you can use to journal this experience.)

**Taking Some Time:** It is true that there may be some things you have to tend to right away, such as attending meetings, or contacting other professionals for appointments. I recommend that you focus only on the most pressing things at this time. While there is a critical window for children to achieve the best outcomes, your process of taking control of this situation, and making informed and deliberate decisions at the beginning of the journey, will have many positive ripples of impact as you move forward. Allow yourself the time to decide how you want to proceed and what kind of SLP would work well with your child. You may even want to develop a sense of what your child responds best to; these criteria may help you evaluate whether an SLP is good match for you and your child. I would caution you to try to stay away from Google and other Internet searching as much as possible until you are under the care of your SLP. Information on the Internet is unregulated and often represents a skewed sample of any particular diagnosis. Reading about worst-case scenarios and other troubling revelations will not help you prepare for the road ahead, and it may actually hold you back by keeping you stuck in fear and dread.

**Find Support:** The parents who seem the most successful at navigating this process are the ones who find their support system early. Identify those people in your life who can be your sounding board, who can allow you to vent, and who can help you stay focused. This may be different people you turn to for different reasons, and that is a good thing. Perhaps your spouse is the one who helps you get things done, but your best friend or minister is the one who allows you to process your emotions without judgment. And your sister is the one who helps you keep yourself focused and lends a hand with your other kids or when you just need a break.

It is important at this point to recognize what you *need*, and to be able to identify those who can easily fill those needs, so that you are not met with frustration when you reach out. This can be a source of conflict in marriages, since men and women process difficult situations so differently, which will be discussed later. You may also find that you resonate most strongly with other parents who are in a similar circumstance; check with your SLP or local agencies to find out about support groups or parent groups that may be available in your area. No one can understand you as well as someone who is facing the same challenges that you are.

As you move through the process, and your child grows up and new challenges present themselves, recognize that your needs and your support system may change as well. Perhaps someone who was critical to your survival early on, when you needed a lot of childcare help, is not needed as much when the child is in full-day school programs. Or, as you develop your skills and savvy as a parent, you are more confident and less reliant on others to process your emotions. What is most important is to be in touch with your own needs and to be bold and direct in your efforts to meet them. Reach out and ask for help in whatever way it is needed, whenever it is needed. When your needs are being met, your child benefits, too.

**Get Organized:** In the beginning, when you are just receiving a diagnosis, you may need to make a list of questions for your physician or other professionals. As you begin to gather information and to get a sense of what you will need to do, many questions will come up. Have a central but portable place to record these, and bring the list with you to your visits with physicians and therapists. Make sure you have space to record key points and information, and a way to retrieve it later. Some parents even audio-record their visits with health care professionals because memory can be faulty, especially when there is a lot of information to process.

The parents that I have worked with over the years have developed some of the most amazing organizational systems I have ever seen. Many parents have identified being organized as one of the key ways they stay on top of all the details and maintain their sanity in the face of so many demands on their time and attention. Being organized is also something that is self-defined. A system that works well for one person may be confusing and overwhelming to another. Tapping into how your brain works to process information, and using that to design your own system will save you a lot of legwork later. Some elements to consider:

- Having *one* calendar where everything is stored. Managing multiple calendars can result in overbooking, missed appointments, and confusion.

- Having a place where everything is stored, with separate files or folders for each professional who works with your child, in date order so it tells a story.
- Having a primary binder or document that has the essentials, including current medications and schedules, allergies, history information, and special instructions. It is especially helpful to have the most critical or common information that everyone asks for in an easy-to-access format that you can easily hand over so you don't spend time filling out forms repetitively. This also helps if your child is medically involved and has many medications; this way you don't have to rely on your memory if you are tired or stressed.
- Having a place for correspondence, organized by professional or insurance carrier, in date order.
- Setting up a place to archive information quarterly or monthly, but where it can still be accessed if needed.
- Given the significant use of technology in 2016, you may want to scan and store things on your hard drive, or use a system like Google Docs or Dropbox to make your information accessible from anywhere.

What is most important is to develop a system early on, to relieve yourself of having to hold too many details in your mind. Further, you need to keep the system updated, which does take some effort. If you need help with this, talk to your SLP. She may have ideas or templates you can use to get started.

## YOUR CHANGING ROLES

*Changing self as parent:* Having a child with any sort of special need requires you to redefine yourself as a parent, and to integrate new aspects or skills into your parenting. First, you may have to redefine your parenting in relation to your work life. If you work outside the home, you may need to adjust your hours or schedule to accommodate therapy appointments and other needs, which may impact your salary or benefits. You may have to change your focus or goals that you had for your career track, or to give up working altogether for a time, while your child's needs are more intense. It is important to recognize and to process what this means for you as a parent and as a person. Parenting a child with communication and behavior challenges can be more intensive and time-consuming that you expected, and it may require more work absences or flexibility in scheduling.

Second, in addition to the changes in your work life, you may also face difficulties in finding appropriate childcare. If your child is more medically involved, or has significant communication and behavior issues, it can be challenging to find childcare providers who are knowledgeable and whom you can trust to take care of your child's needs. Extended family members who may have provided care in the past may feel overwhelmed and fearful about being responsible for your child. Even for children who have isolated speech or language issues, extra effort and skill is required to keep them from being frustrated and on track. Take your time in finding providers whom you feel comfortable with, and who have the necessary skills and training, or who are willing to learn from you what your child needs and how to be a member of your team.

Third, you may be learning a whole new language. Whether you are in the neonatal intensive care unit (NICU), and surrounded by doctors and nurses, or in early intervention (EI), surrounded by therapists and educators, chances are it seems like everyone around you speaks in acronyms. You will need to learn the vocabulary of your child's diagnosis, as well as the terminology around its treatment. It is important that you *ask* if you do not know what something means, because your ability to advocate for your child depends on your understanding of the process and the people working with your child. As therapists, we are so used to speaking in jargon that we do not even notice when we are doing it. Sometimes it takes a parent's question to prompt us to tune in to your needs, so that what we are saying can be understood and processed. You may even want to ask your SLP for a list of vocabulary and acronyms that you might encounter around your child's treatment. You can refer back to chapter 2 for some common terminology.

Finally, you will most likely be developing a whole new set of skills and roles. In addition to all the normal parenting decisions that you have to make, you may be asked to play the part of:

- Lifeline: for children with communication issues, you will likely be their interpreter as the one who understands them best. They may be more dependent on you than a typical child and require more assistance.
- Detective or research analyst: You will likely be looking into different techniques, reading about treatment protocols, or finding technology that might help your child.
- Care coordinator: Overseeing all the professionals who work with your child, often in the absence of communication. You are responsible for making sure that no one is working at cross purposes with others, and managing appointments and therapy sessions around the rest of your family obligations.
- Advocate: This is the role that is most crucial to your child's well-being. You will learn to understand the federal and state laws that apply to your child's education and care, and you will learn to advocate for what your child needs, no matter what the setting or the professional involved. You know your child better than anyone else, and you know what you and your child need. No one else is better equipped to negotiate with doctors and therapists on your child's behalf. Find a local resource where you can learn about the laws that govern the kinds of services and supports your child may be *entitled to* by law.

I have seen many parents take on this role in particular with gusto. For some parents, this even becomes an avocation, and something they reach out to help other families with once their own child's needs are met and he is progressing well in treatment and school. This is a role that comes easily to some parents, and given the right guidance and information, such parent advocates are a powerful source of support for their own child, and other children with special needs.

## CHANGING SELF AS SPOUSE

In addition to changes in your identity as a parent, you may face changes in your marriage when raising a child with special needs. For some families, children have short-term difficulties that resolve, while others face lifelong disabilities and challenges that will evolve over time. Both can and do have an impact on a marriage.

One of the things that is the most striking to me, and that I see most often, is how men and women process difficult situations so differently. Whether it is processing the grief of having a child with some sort of special need or navigating family celebrations, men and women process their emotions differently, and communicate so divergently, that awareness and understanding of this can go a long way to easing conflicts. In *broad general terms*, fathers tend to focus on their emotions in private and may withdraw when feeling something intense. Mothers, who generally like to process their feelings verbally over time, can misinterpret this as lack of concern or a lack of emotional availability. In addition, fathers sometimes prefer to focus on logistics and taking care of financial matters, which they can control; however, this may mean that they are away from the home more often or for longer hours. As, perhaps, now the sole provider for the family with increased financial considerations, fathers may focus intently on that responsibility, sometimes to the exclusion of participating in meetings or appointments or supporting their spouse.

In contrast, mothers may want to talk about their feelings and their challenges and to explore options. Mothers may end up bearing the lion's share of caregiving, as well as navigating therapy appointments and doctor visits on their own. This can lead to feelings of resentment and burnout, as the time and effort (physical and mental) can be punishing.

## Case Examples

Jaden was twenty months old when he came to see me for the first time. He had limited play skills and no speech or language skills beyond crying. He was clearly frustrated, and Mom and Dad were, too. They were afraid of what would happen to their son and wondered if he would ever speak. Jaden was due to be evaluated by a developmental medicine team, and we discussed the possibility that he might be diagnosed with autism. Regardless of that diagnosis, he had a severe communication deficit and hard work ahead with developing speech and language skills. As we began to work together, Mom focused on participating in her sessions with me, learning everything she could, and carrying over every recommendation I gave her. She also used our sessions to process some of her feelings and fears about her son and her marriage. While Mom was focused on working with me, Dad was withdrawn. He was focused on all that he thought his son might never be and the things they might never do together. He did not attend sessions with me and openly wondered if there would be any progress. This was obviously a strain in their relationship, and for a time, they could not help one another. As Jaden began to make progress, and to connect with each of his parents, Dad slowly began to work through his fears. He began to ask questions and even attended a few sessions on his own. My office felt like a safe space for Dad to ask his own questions and explore his own ability to connect with and help Jaden, and so he began to participate more. The more that Dad participated, and felt successful, the more Jaden's parents were able to come back together around his needs, and his skills began to blossom. Today, Jaden is a happy, energetic kindergartener whose skills are above age level in several areas. His story shows you how his parents reacted quite differently to his challenges, but with help and support and time, they were each able to contribute in positive ways to his growth.

Sawyer was twenty-five months old when he first came to see me. He had one or two words, but he did not use them consistently. He was the beloved fourth child in a stable family whose older children were all ahead of the game developmentally. Sawyer was beginning to get frustrated at being unable to keep up with his siblings and never getting what he wanted. He did not seem as happy as his siblings. He tended to withdraw and not even try to communicate. Mom and Dad were both employed full time but worked different hours from each other so that they could handle all the childcare needs. Sawyer's parents reported feeling a bit surprised by his communication issues since none of their other children had a problem in this area. They both had a lot of questions and wanted to do whatever was necessary to support his progress. They also had very different styles of interacting with Sawyer. Mom was animated and fun, and jumped right in to playing on the floor and using the communication techniques I taught her. Dad was very quiet and was unsure of how to play with Sawyer. He seemed surprised by the things he saw Sawyer do when interacting with me. Over time, Dad learned how to be a good language facilitator, and Mom told me she saw the difference in their interactions immediately. Sawyer made rapid progress with his skills, and he went on to "graduate" after about six months.

Both of these case examples show how, as parents, you may need different types and levels of support from your SLP. You may need modeling of a technique and some support and feedback, and you are good to go. Your spouse may need more time and more help with developing good language-facilitation skills. However, whether you and your spouse start out in the same place is less important than that you end up there.

In addition to how they process emotions, spouses can differ in their views and ability to manage several areas, including:

- Financial matters: Who decides what money is spent? What expenses must be sacrificed? Who determines whether a new therapy or activity gets added to the schedule? How does the impact of copays and other medical expenses affect the other kids in the house? How compatible are your financial goals?
- Caregiving: Who can provide care for the child? What special training is needed? What strategies and behavior techniques do your child's caregivers need to know?
- Extended family concerns: How do you tell people about your child's diagnosis? How do you manage your child at family gatherings? How will you take advice and information from family? (In my experience, the answer is "with a grain of salt.")
- Time management: How do you preserve time for yourselves as a couple? Make time for other kids? Hobbies? Who gets that night out when you are both burnt out and tired?

There is conventional wisdom that parents of children with special needs divorce at a higher rate than those with typical children. In my clinical experience, this is not necessarily true. In doing research for this book, I found that many of the studies that report such findings are poorly supported by research and lack the necessary rigor to be considered.[2] This may be reassuring for you, as adding another layer of complexity through divorce may seem unthinkable. What is true in my experience is that whatever issues were present before the birth of a child with special needs remain. They may even be magnified. However, with the proper support, and with an understanding of how your partner is processing things, you can come together and create a stronger, healthier, and more vibrant partnership that supports your whole family. Or you can collapse and break apart. As with most things in life, it depends on the meaning you give it, and how you face a tough situation. A bit of understanding and compassion can go a long way, and learning to communicate in productive ways can make a huge difference in the growth and evolution of your marriage. This may be an area where counseling can be helpful.

## THE CHANGING FAMILY UNIT

Just as you and your spouse are going through an adjustment, so are your other children. There may be confusion and fear as they try to understand what is happening with their sibling, or they may be feeling left out and resentful that they no longer get as much of your attention. There can be both positive and negative outcomes, even within the same family. Some issues to consider:

- Distribution of time: Fairness plays into a lot of parent's feelings. When one child requires a lot of time or intensive care, other siblings may feel slighted and resent their brother or sister. They may also have to sacrifice some of their hobbies or activities due to financial burdens or time constraints.
- Siblings of children with challenges often have to grow up quickly. They may have to be on their own more frequently or spend a lot of time going to appointments. There is often less time to just relax at home, have play dates, and quiet family time.
- Having one or more children with challenges definitely impacts the family's ability to pick up and go do things on weekends or go on vacations. Perhaps there are extra appointments or therapy practice that needs to be done, or simply a need to catch up on housework. There may also be considerations for a child with challenges to not be out in the community, such as frequent meltdowns or other behavioral issues.
- Fairness also plays into behavior management and expectations for behavior. As children with communication challenges grow

up, their developmental level may be well below their age; thus, they are not expected to play by the same rules as their siblings. This can lead to resentment and acting out toward the child with communication issues, due to siblings' lack of understanding.

- On the positive side, siblings of children with communication and developmental challenges can also develop extraordinary compassion and empathy. They frequently become advocates for their sibling, and may even stand up for other vulnerable kids in school or in the neighborhood. Some siblings are also great caregivers, learning sign language or other things they can do to help out. Some siblings end up choosing a career in a helping profession because of their early experiences. They certainly learn to love deeply and to see the goodness in others.

How a sibling responds is in large part due to how he or she understands what is happening in the family, and how he or she is asked to cultivate the traits that define helpful and empathetic tendencies. Making time for typical siblings, recognizing their contributions, and keeping them updated can go a long way to making the positive outweigh the negative.

*Extended family concerns*: Our family of origin gives us many things: our eye color, our temperament, and even our beliefs about money. Our spouse's family gave them the same. And in many cases, the two can be quite different. Thus, our extended family can be a source of strength, hope, love, and support, or a source of stress and conflict. This depends on several factors.

- Understanding of the situation: If there is not a family history of special needs, extended family may have a lack of awareness or understanding of the diagnosis or how to care for you or your child. I have heard parents talk countless times about how often something is said in an attempt to be helpful, but is instead received as hurtful or intrusive. In contrast, other extended families go out of their way to learn, to keep up with therapy progress, and always try to encourage you.
- Respect for parenting style: Every parent has their reasons for making the choices that they do. In fact, our style of parenting is often in response to how we were parented. This might mean

doing the opposite of what you experienced, or imitating a style you felt was effective and appropriate. When you are parenting *in front of the ones who parented you* (or your spouse), it can be rife with opportunities for misunderstanding and conflict. You may need to spend time educating your family about your child's particular challenges and why you are using specific strategies to help your child get better. Sadly, sometimes you have to make hard choices about family gatherings and who is able to support you and your child.

- Participation in family gatherings: Depending on your child's needs, it may be difficult to attend large family gatherings. This may be due to your child's tendency to be easily overwhelmed in crowds or unfamiliar places, or because of the onslaught of advice and questions that you may face. In contrast, family gatherings may be a time when you can relax and others can step in to give you a break, and when you can sit back in the safe space that is your family.
- View of disability/faith: Just as each family has its own history and style, each family has a different view on disability. Some families and religious traditions view having a child with a disability as a curse or punishment and may seek to determine what you may have done to make this happen. You or your child may be viewed with pity, suspicion, or contempt. In contrast, others view such life experiences as blessings or opportunities, with your child being viewed as a special messenger who can teach everyone an important lesson about being human. Many families fall somewhere in between. Your family may also have a different view from your spouse's family. Learning to let hurtful comments go when moving between families is an important skill.
- Family roles: Whenever Thanksgiving rolls around, it seems like everyone gets transported back in time. Gathering and interacting with families can also mean playing out old dramas from when you were much younger. Yet somehow, even when you are married and dealing with your own life issues, the family table can somehow make you twelve years old again. Or you witness your very confident, in-control spouse, revert to being a shy kid who refused to speak up for himself and now gets steamrolled in family discussions. This can be disconcerting if you don't realize what is hap-

pening. Your relationships with your siblings can also be affected when you have a child with special needs. If you are competitive, there may be feelings of resentment if you are jealous of your sister's typical kids. Or maybe your brother can't stop talking about the vacations and fancy things he is doing that you can't afford right now because you have a mountain of medical debt. This also applies to your role as a son or daughter. How your parent viewed you as a child or teen can color his or her ability to see you as capable, strong, and organized in the face of extraordinary circumstances.

When considering all of these factors, it is important to stay in touch with your feelings. As discussed earlier, your ability to connect with and process your emotions plays an important part in your physical and mental health. Being honest with yourself and your spouse, keeping the lines of communication open, and being gentle and compassionate with everyone involved, will leave open the possibility for great healing and new understanding and perspective.

Having a child with communication issues can be challenging in both expected and unexpected ways. In my practice, parents often report a range of emotional challenges, including but not limited to the following:

- feeling exhausted and overwhelmed;
- feeling separated from their spouse emotionally;
- feeling stretched too thin, unable to meet everyone's needs;
- feeling stymied by a lack of understanding from others;
- feeling undermined by well-meaning relatives and friends.

There is no one, right way to navigate a life experience such as this. Every person and every family unit finds their way through it. Some find many blessings while others find only obstacles. And know this: Every person's journey is perfect as it is. That may be difficult to read, but when you look back on this time later in your life, it is more likely that you will relate how much you gained than how much you lost. Here are some things that may help you on your path.

*Finding the new normal*: There is a point with every family that I work with where something subtle changes, and there is a settling into a routine. Perhaps a medical crisis passes, or the routine gets easier to manage. Either way, families find a way to marshal their resources and settle into the reality of daily life. For some families, this happens early on, while others take several years to reach that place. Whatever you are struggling with right now, know that it will most likely change. It will evolve, and so will you. The feelings of overwhelm might still be there, but you will be more confident in your ability to manage them. Or you may make changes to your schedule that allow your spouse to participate more. What is most important is to recognize and honor where you are and to ask for what you need.

*Resolving conflicts*: It is important to minimize the sources of stress in your life, for many reasons. Do not allow conflict with your spouse, parent, or sibling to add to your emotional burdens. Seek help as needed, or just open your heart and listen to your partner. Talk deeply about what you need and work to find solutions that will uplift both of you.

*Making time*: Time seems to be in short supply these days. It is critical that you make the effort to find time for your spouse, for your children, and for yourself. Take the time to prioritize what is most important right now, recognizing that this can and will change over time. Do you need to let something go? This might be a weekly obligation, an extra activity, or that twelfth therapy appointment in a week. Embrace the concept of Good Enough, and release the need for Perfection. As someone who has been chasing Perfection for many years, I have come to realize that it is the elusive unicorn that can steal your presence from the moment, and the joy from your life. Get help with what you can, and release the rest. It will free you up to focus on the things that really matter to you.

*Changing your definition of success*: Each family defines success for themselves. Maybe having your child healthy enough to go through the holidays without a serious meltdown is meaningful. Or perhaps having a schedule that gives you time to play with your child, or have a family outing once a month, is what you want. Part of prioritizing is determining what will make you feel most productive and happy.

*Keeping yourself in sight*: This is critical. Go ahead and make an asterisk next to this point. This may be the most important piece because if you are not at your best, everything fails. In my experience, it is usually the mother who is most involved in the day-to-day running of the house and managing everyone's schedules. Women often serve as the emotional center and the leaders of their families. (This is not meant to underestimate the dedication and efforts of very involved fathers.) In order to do this, to care deeply about yourself, you must support yourself in body, mind, and spirit.

- Physical self-care might be getting a massage, engaging in regular exercise, taking supplements, and getting enough sleep. It cannot be said enough how important it is to get enough good-quality sleep so that you stay healthy and vital, to be present for everyone.
- Mental and emotional self-care might include things like processing your emotions, getting out with friends, or staying off Google for a while. It is important to get out of deficit focus and recharge by having some fun and release.
- Spiritual self-care means having some sort of spiritual practice, from meditation to a regular church routine. Beyond that, however, it means engaging your creativity and doing things that bring you joy and peace.

They say that you can't pour anything from a broken cup. While it may seem overwhelming at times to make the time for yourself, making the effort pays off. I often hear mothers say they can't take care of themselves because they can't be that selfish. It is not selfish to *care for the one who cares for everyone else*. It is exactly the opposite. You set the tone, you set the pace, and you provide the example of how things can be done. Reach out and get the support you need in the way that works for you. Everyone will benefit in the long run.

# 8

# FINDING THE NEW NORMAL

## Moving Forward and Taking Charge

If you have read the previous chapter, you have already started on your journey as a parent of a child with communication challenges. You have taken some time to process your emotions, you have asked many questions, and you have worked on developing a system of keeping information and appointments straight. Hopefully, you have also been taking good care of yourself and making good communication with your partner a priority. With these new facts in mind, we can now begin to talk about some of the skills you will begin to develop in the next stage.

I developed the following list of skills and traits by watching thousands of parents over the years, and by asking some of them directly what they felt were the most important lessons they had to learn on their journey. The ones presented below are by no means exhaustive; you may find many more that are true for you. It is my hope that reading about these traits will give you something to aspire to, to reach for, and to cultivate.

### SKILLS THAT CAN BE DEVELOPED

*Advocacy*: As we discussed in the previous chapter, you will become an advocate for your child. This role may also be played by teachers, therapists, and others who love your child, but no one will be better than you at putting a laser focus on your child's needs and what is best for her. Developing this skill can happen quickly, or slowly over a long period of time. You can begin by reading about special education law, knowing your rights, and talking to other parents. In Massachusetts, where I practice, parents can also access help, information, and referrals for advocacy services from the Federation for Children with Special Needs.[1] What is most important for you is to think carefully about what you already know: *your child*. You know his strengths and weaknesses, his personality, and his likes and dislikes. Your SLP can also be a good source of information and a resource for thinking about what your child needs in school, in community groups, or at home.

*Communication*: This skill was also discussed at length in the previous chapter as it relates to your marriage and your family. Good communication skills are also critical in dealing with doctors, therapists, and teachers. It is important to have open, non-adversarial dialogue with those who are entrusted with your child's care. You want to work with professionals who encourage you to ask questions, who listen to you and your concerns, and who want to partner with you to help your child develop. Although emotions can run high, it is best to strategize with professionals when you have a clear idea of what you want to address, as well as what you are looking for. As an SLP, I have had a few experiences where a parent came to me very upset about something in their child's treatment plan. Perhaps it was the way I corrected the child in a session, or the way I addressed a behavior. Of course, I always want to know when there are questions, or when something is amiss. However, the hardest of those conversations happen when it seems that the parent does not have a sense of what they want: Changes in goals? More therapy time? Better communication with home and school? To be heard because you are having a tough day?

Ironically, communication is both easier and more challenging than when I started practicing in 1994. The realities of caseloads and service delivery were very different then and often allowed for professionals to meet regularly and discuss the plan for a particular child. In early intervention (EI), teams met weekly or monthly so everyone was on the same page. All of those realities are quite different now with managed care, and with higher productivity and caseload requirements in hospitals and schools. It is harder to get everyone together to talk, since the days of a professional are often stretched quite thin. On the other hand, technology such as e-mail and texting make people more readily available outside of regular business hours. Although these activities are governed by the rules of the Healthcare Insurance Portability and Accountability Act (HIPAA), the law that governs how your private information is collected and used, it can be helpful to have more options to communicate.

*Negotiation*: You will often find yourself in situations where a professional or team will present a plan for your approval. It might be an Individualized Education Plan (IEP) for your child's school, or a medical plan to treat some aspect of your child's condition. It is important to think of these presentations as the "opening bid" in a negotiation. It can be challenging to do this when the underlying message is, "We are the professionals. Accept the plan we are giving you because we know better." Remember that you are the foremost expert on your child. You are the one who can read your child's subtle expressions and know what they mean. You are the one who has been to every appointment and has a sense of what each professional's plan is. If you can approach these conversations as you might any other negotiation, you will be able to keep in mind that it can't be a zero-sum game. Everyone has to feel that they are walking away having made an impact. If you have the negotiation mindset, you will also project an air of calm, and you will be able to communicate your clear vision. It may also be helpful to decide ahead of time which items are absolutes, and which ones you could be flexible about. Remember, too, that your right as the parent includes calling a meeting of your team whenever you feel that it is needed.

If something is added to your plan that you are unsure will benefit your child, but you are taking a recommendation to try something new, put in the plan that you want a meeting in four weeks. That way, you won't have to ask later for a meeting, and you will be able to evaluate whether the plan is working when there is ample time to change it.

*Organization*: It is worth mentioning this skill again, even though it was covered in the previous chapter. Parents have told me over and over again how much more in control they feel when they have a system that makes it easy to find information and to track what all the various professionals are telling them. Again, create a system that works for you, is flexible, and exists in more than one place. Put an electronic copy on a flash drive, make archive copies, or keep one in the Cloud. No matter where you are, or what happens, you will be able to access all your information.

*Time management*: This skill was also covered in the previous chapter, but it is worth mentioning again. It is important to identify your priorities and use your time accordingly. When you know what is most important to you, such as being present with your child in therapy sessions or having family dinner with all your children, it becomes easier to make decisions and resolve time conflicts. Something you are being asked to do is either in line with your priorities or it is not. As a therapist, I sometimes have to honor a parent's wish to miss a session because they are focusing on something else that day. Even though the parent may be very dedicated to their child's treatment, sometimes they need to be present for a typical sibling's performance at school, or they need a mental health day with their spouse or child.

*Behavior management*: This is another key skill that evolves over time. It may also require some support or education from a teacher or therapist that you trust, to show you how to implement strategies. Children with speech and language issues often need more supports and prompts in place to maintain their behavior while completing a task. Children with challenging sensory needs may also need certain kinds of stimulation or activities to help them maintain a calm state. It is important that whatever behavior plan you develop is appropriate to your child's level of understanding and that it is consistently followed. Everyone in the child's life, including therapists and grandparents or caregivers, needs to follow the same routine when addressing behavior. When developing a behavior plan, there are a few factors to consider:

- 
  - What is one specific behavior that I want to address? It may be hitting or biting that can affect their placement in school or peer relationships; alternatively, it may be a self-injurious behavior that poses a safety risk.
  - Determine what the function of the behavior is. One of the most salient moments of my career came a few months after starting my residency, while attending my first annual convention. I attended a presentation by a clinician discussing behavior management. He said, "Behavior is *always* communication." It has impacted my entire career. When I speak with

parents about challenging behaviors, I always encourage them to be a detective and determine what the child is trying to communicate through the use of that behavior. Sometimes, they are communicating that they are bored or frustrated, or that they just want your attention. Understanding the purpose for their behavior may guide you in a completely different direction and allow you to connect with your child on a much deeper level.

- If you have identified the problem behavior, determine what you are trying to develop in its place. It may be that you want to encourage asking for help or a break, or to learn to verbalize difficult feelings without physically acting out.

- Determine what the consequence will be for exhibiting the problem behavior. Will your child go to time-out? What will that routine be? Will they lose TV time or a physical possession such as an iPad? What is the reward for demonstrating the new behavior? What language or prompts will you use to talk about the behavior?

- Be sure to outline how you will know when the behavior is changed, and how you will measure that change, so that you can begin to provide supports that allow your child to use the new behavior more independently. You may also want to move on to addressing the next problematic behavior at that time.

- Sometimes ignoring a behavior goes a long way toward eliminating it. For some common behaviors, such as dropping food off their high chair, or screeching, your child may be seeking your attention. She wants to interact with you but lacks the communication skills necessary to initiate and sustain interaction. At this stage, your child cannot differentiate between positive attention and negative attention (scolding, etc.). In fact, sometimes a young child interprets negative attention as an invitation to play a silly game where you make funny faces and use a funny voice. In these situations, where safety is not at risk, allow yourself to walk away or just avoid eye contact. For children at a younger developmental stage, the withdrawal of your social attention can be an effective deterrent. She learns quickly that when she engages in those behaviors, you turn away; this helps reduce or eliminate those behaviors in a simple way without fancy behavior plans. One caveat, though—children learn very quickly how to get your attention. And following through on behavior management techniques is an important part of your development as well as your child's. Having a sense that you can manage your child's behavior in any situation provides comfort and confidence, and will allow you to tackle other challenges as well.

One final skill that I encourage you to develop is your *intuition*. For some, this comes easily, while for others, it may take some time. For our purposes, developing your intuition means learning to trust yourself to make decisions, and that *you know what you know*. As a parent, you often know early on that there is a problem with your child. You know when a teacher or therapist is connecting with your child and understands and cares for him or her. You also know when something feels amiss, and you are uncomfortable about a program, professional, or situation. It cannot be overemphasized how important it is to follow your intuition. If you have questions, ask. If you have concerns, raise them. Perhaps your opening up the lines of communication will lead you to a better understanding of a professional's motivations or techniques. Or, your fears might be well founded and then you can take the steps you need to correct the situation. Follow your intuition, and your child will always benefit.

The next part of this chapter will discuss some of the internal traits that you will want to cultivate to be a successful parent and advocate.

*Confidence*: This follows from educating yourself about your child's condition or diagnosis, being organized and focused, and following your intuition. Recognizing your own value, and the essential role you play in your child's development and habilitation is critical to your child's success. I often see parents who struggle with decisions about some aspect of their child's life. They ask me for an opinion because I am the "professional." True, I have many years experience in working with children who have speech and language issues, and I may have seen similar situations before. However, most parents know the right answer for their child, but they hesitate to make it out of fear that it will be wrong. There are very few decisions that you make that can't be undone if it turns out in a way that is not in your child's best interest, and more often than not, you are right on target. Partnering with professionals you trust can help you develop confidence, and even to practice/role-play situations where you feel less capable of communicating confidently.

*Flexibility*: Just as we are a reflection of our parents, our children are a reflection of us—the best and the worst. Many children with special needs, and especially language delays, make a strong bid for control in situations where they feel uncomfortable. You may do the same thing when going into a meeting with your child's educational team, or into an important medical appointment. Learning to be flexible allows you to step away from situations that just don't warrant your time or energy, or to step outside your comfort zone and allow your child to try something new. Flexibility also allows you to negotiate, and to stay true to your priorities. If flexibility is a challenge for you, you may want to work with a friend, family member, or professional that you trust to look at the various perspectives in a situation and see how your view changes with the information they provide. Allowing yourself to let go of the little things and focus on the bigger picture will also support your mental and emotional health.

*Acceptance*: In the previous chapter, we discussed some of the stages you may experience when faced with a diagnosis for your child. Grief is a primary one, and it has its own stages as well.[2] Acceptance is the final stage, when you have faced your loss, moved through all of its aspects, and come to a place of peace with your new normal. Although it may never be what you hoped for or expected, you find yourself able to talk about your child's challenges with less emotion, or you find yourself beginning to focus on the positives in your child's life and personality rather than just their problems or deficits. This is an important trait to acquire because it often signals the beginning of a new chapter in your life. Perhaps you begin advocating for your child in a new way, or you may even have a sense of renewed purpose in your own life. Acceptance does not imply that you do not have pain or frustration, only that you see your circumstances from a higher place and no longer feel quite so overwhelmed by things.

*Patience*: This is one I hear about a lot from parents. Who has time to be patient, right? Waiting for therapists, waiting for your child to acquire that new skill, waiting for that quiet time at the end of the week. . . . It all takes a toll on us daily. Learning to be patient means cultivating the part of us that knows there is a bigger plan and that all is taken care of in time. It also means remembering that things happen in cycles and that sometimes, just when you think your child is hopelessly stuck, they learn a new skill or make a leap in their development.

*A sense of humor*: This is another one I often hear about from many parents. Sometimes you just have to laugh. It won't always come easy, but it will come in time. Maybe one day you notice that your child is playing a silly game with you, or you have one of those "I can't believe that really happened" moments in the grocery store. Either way, over time, you can develop an appreciation of the subtle things, such as your child's smile that can brighten your day no matter what you are dealing with.

*Perspective*: This is a trait that develops over years, not weeks. Learning to view your child's development in layers and cycles, you gradually become aware of how things go and that the beginning of any new cycle brings back old feelings and calls on old skills yet again. You also learn that you have faced similar challenges in the past, that things have a way of working themselves out, and that you can always call on those friends, family, or professionals whom you know you can trust. I also see this in the way that parents slowly begin to define their child by abilities and personality, rather than by a list of their deficits. And when this happens for you, you also begin to demand the same from the professionals who work with your child. This is to everyone's benefit, as seeing your child for the *whole* person that they are can sometimes help integrate many different pieces. We will talk further about perspective in the final chapter of this book.

## DRIVING THE THERAPY PROCESS AS TEAM LEADER

As you are developing the skills discussed above, and certainly once you have mastered them, you are prepared to take your rightful place as the *leader* of your child's development and treatment program. You can cast off the false elevation of professionals and seek their genuine input as equals. You can make decisions and set expectations for those who work with you in ways that benefit your child, and you as parent.

One of the frustrations I hear most often is that parents receive input from many diverse people and that there are usually conflicts between professionals. There may be disagreement about the diagnosis, the most appropriate goals, or how to address behavior. Frequently, I hear parents relate that everyone on the team gives homework, and every professional thinks their specialty is the *most* important one that should be focused on. While there is some information available about developmental progression, and there may be some skills that need to be worked on before others, it should not fall to you as parent to navigate that alone. This is where communication becomes critical, and requiring team members to connect in a meeting can be helpful. Again, the use of technologies allows people to meet virtually, after business hours, or from anywhere. When there are conflicts, ask that they be settled and that a plan be developed. Each professional can present their information, and a decision can be made based on *all* the information.

Professionals do the best they can with what they know, and with good intentions—to help your child. However, you are the one who is with your child 24/7 and can provide that cohesion and demand that communication. In the absence of such parental leadership, professionals will continue to do their job in good faith and may miss the opportunity to be more holistic in their approach. Don't be afraid to advocate for your child in requesting that everyone communicate, and that everyone find consensus with how to approach a particular question or situation.

Helping to find common ground and resolving team conflicts is an unfortunate part of managing a team. There are different approaches and perspectives in the diagnosis and treatment of most childhood disorders. Trust that you have the ability to make decisions about your child's plan, even if that means removing a team member who is unable to reach consensus or who is unwilling to work with others. Remember—*you know what you know*!

As mentioned above, parents are often challenged to complete daily or weekly homework with their child by most therapists. This is grounded in an understanding of learning theory, which teaches us that what we practice gets stronger. From a brain perspective, we know that what "fires often gets wired," meaning that when neurons fire, it strengthens existing networks and activates new networks of cooperating neurons. When we engage in a behavior repetitively, whether it is a body movement or a speech sound, it becomes more and more engrained and then automatic. However, what professionals don't know is the context that you are embedding all this homework in. Perhaps they don't know that you are working sixty hours a week because you have missed so many days, or you are so tired you don't have it in you every day to push your child's limits after a full day of school or therapies.

This is a tricky situation. As an SLP, I give homework. I talk to parents about the importance of practice and how it makes the overall therapy process shorter and more effective. I have parents who faithfully execute every exercise and those who struggle to even get the homework folder out to the car, and every shade in between. In my practice, I try to focus on ways that they can target our goals within their daily activities and routines. After all, speech and language are happening all the time! Chances are, you can find ways to covertly target goals for specific speech sounds, or to incorporate something into bath time that fulfills the requirement for practice. The nice thing about those activities is that the child is working on thinking about their goal in a natural communication context, and not just the structured practice we focus on in our sessions. I have also seen parents come up with very creative games on their own. I encourage parents to use the materials I give as a starting place, a source of words with their target sound, but not to worry when they don't do sit-down practice. And there are some weeks when no real "practice" happens at all. While that may not be ideal from an SLP perspective, my understanding and empathy around the whole picture supports their trust in me and fosters my positive relationships with families. Allow your SLP to support you so that you can get back to practice as soon as possible, rather than turning away from it due to negative feelings and experiences.

If you find yourself having trouble working practice into your day, ask the therapists or teachers involved for help. Be honest with your SLP about any challenges around homework that come up. We can only be helpful if we understand the whole picture. Brainstorm together some ways that you can fit practice into things you already do so you don't feel like you have to set aside a separate time to practice. Let us help you develop a plan that works for you and moves your child in the direction of progress.

The same goes for therapy sessions. Often, in the early years, parents want to maximize therapy hours, and they seek to get everything they can for their child. This can sometimes result in stress and overwhelm for everyone. As things move along, and particularly for those children who have longer-term disabilities, your view on this may change. It is perfectly acceptable to periodically reevaluate your child's total plan and to assess each program or therapy to determine if changes should be made. Perhaps you schedule fewer sessions per week, or you let one therapy go if it is not as effective. Referring back to your identified priorities and staying true to what is most important will help guide your decisions about these issues. I am not advocating giving up on your child's treatment, but rather identifying those areas that are positive and uplifting and those that do not support your well-being or your child's. If you feel frustrated about a particular therapy, chances are your child does, too. Remembering that life is more than the sum of your therapy parts, and that sometimes the best thing you can do for your family is to let go of something that is not working, can be a positive step.

## ALTERNATIVE APPROACHES

These days, there are many different ways to approach complex conditions such as autism. For every conventional and well-known program, there are several lesser known alternative treatments, with new ones showing up all the time. As the parent and team leader, you may want to investigate some of these approaches at various points in your child's life, especially if traditional therapies are not working as you had hoped.

The first thing to know is that some of these approaches are untested and have no scientific research to support them. For some treatments, there is no safety risk, and all you may lose is some of your time and money. However, other treatments may pose a risk to your child's safety, such as untested supplements, radical movement therapies, or other programs that promise amazing results in a short time.

Before you try any such treatment, it is important to ask questions about how the treatment was developed and by whom, and what theory of development or dysfunction the treatment is based on. It is also important to know if there have been any adverse outcomes from the treatment, and how much of an investment you are being asked to make. Unfortunately, there are many people out there who are vested not in your child's best interest but, rather, in making money off of vulnerable parents who are seeking answers and help for their child. Always use your intuition and carefully evaluate any new approach before you try it with your child. Remember, there is no magic bullet to cure communication issues or autism. There is no replacement for well-provided, scientifically based treatment.

In my own practice, I use two "alternative" approaches, Reiki and craniosacral therapy (CST) to augment and expand my traditional SLP work. I have come to use these two modalities because they have no adverse physical or developmental side affects and because you can tell functionally fairly quickly if they have a positive impact. Both Reiki and CST have a basis in medical understanding of the body and have ongoing research into their effectiveness, safety, and use. When it seems as though a particular family might benefit from one or both of these approaches, I offer parents information and reading material. We talk about why I think it would be helpful and discuss any answer questions. If a parent wishes to try one or both of these approaches, then we move forward.

It is worth noting here that for some parents, these kinds of approaches may seem way out of the box, or even a little "woo-woo." I admit that it took me quite some time as a clinician with my background in medical SLP to invite parents to explore these modalities with me. Healthy skepticism is welcome because you need to be discerning when it comes to what you do with your child. You can feel free to skip this section of the book if it feels as though it is not for you. However, if you feel drawn to read more, and then consider some of the clinical experiences I have had using these techniques with children.

Reiki is a gentle hands-on energy modality that is based on the idea that you can tap into and channel universal energy through the hands. The practice of Reiki was developed in Japan and came to the United States in the 1950s.[3] Practitioners are attuned by a Reiki Master, who opens the energy system of a person's body, allowing that person to direct this energy to themselves and others. Once you are attuned, you are taught to feel the flow of this energy in others and to help facilitate this energy flow. It is thought that where energy becomes blocked in the body, disease or illness can show up. By facilitating a return of uninterrupted energy flow, you can release physical and emotional problems in the body.

In my experience, Reiki can be helpful for children who need to experience positive touch. For some children, the world can seem like a scary place, and one where they cannot express themselves easily or understand what is happening. Using Reiki (which involves placing the hands on or just above the skin) promotes relaxation and rest, which also allows the body to heal. Reiki is being used more and more frequently in medical settings and hospitals. Cancer patients and children undergoing surgery or medical procedures are being offered Reiki before, during, or after their procedures. The research now being done indicates many positive benefits, from a lower level of pain and need for pain medication to relaxation and lower blood pressure, shorter hospital stays, and better wound healing.[4] I recommend Reiki for children who have had a lot of invasive or unpleasant medical procedures, or for those who seem uncomfortable in their skin and need a gentle hand. Parents are always present and can always refuse this adjunct to traditional SLP work.

The other modality I use is craniosacral therapy (CST). This is a body of work developed by Dr. John Upledger, an osteopath. The main goal of CST is to normalize the function of the nervous system, which drives everything else in development and life. By allowing the nervous system to self-correct, it is thought that we can encourage whole body healing. CST is provided by trained therapists who use pressure equivalent to five grams, or the weight of a nickel. Practitioners are taught how to tap into the flow of cerebrospinal fluid to assess the health and integrity of various body systems. We then use a series of techniques designed to facilitate the body's own wisdom in healing itself. We often speak of the Inner Wisdom or Inner Physician that resides in all of us. Tapping into that body wisdom can correct some issues that arise from compression somewhere in the system. See the resources section of this book for where to find more information about CST.

I typically recommend CST in addition to traditional SLP in a few circumstances. First, when there is a known neurological diagnosis or issue. If we know that there is something atypical about brain development, we may be able to support self-correction before more serious deficits manifest. Second, I usually recommend CST for children who have significant difficulty in sensory processing and self-regulation. For these children, their world can be overwhelming and scary. CST provides a way for them to deeply relax and to regroup from the stresses in their lives. Finally, I may recommend CST for a child who has a known structural issue, such as vocal nodules, tongue-tie or recurrent ear infections. Using CST in these situations may support a gentle release of the body conditions that perpetuate the problem and support the work of traditional medicine. It is important to note that I use these alternative approaches as an adjunct and not a replacement for my traditional SLP work.

## Case Examples

Zander is a nine-year-old boy who started working with me at four years of age, due to multiple speech and language issues. He had apraxia, mild autism, and significant language delays. Zander also had difficulty with sensory processing and attention. He frequently seemed disorganized and overwhelmed, and he had frequent headaches. We decided to try CST with him several years ago to see how he responded. Usually, Zander received CST after his regular speech session where we worked on his communication and language goals. Zander had a lot of compression in his cranial base (the base of the head) and in the temporal bones, just above the ears. He also had tension in his frontal bone, which makes up the forehead. Using CST has provided him with many benefits over the years. He has fewer headaches, and he is generally calmer. Zander is often deeply relaxed on the massage table, where he reclines to receive CST, giving his nervous system a much-needed rest. One of the reasons I wanted to use CST with Zander is that I believed it would make him more available for learning and benefiting from the traditional SLP work I offered. When he was disorganized, and unable to make sense of the world around him, he was not able to learn new skills or retain information. By CST's facilitating his nervous system's ability to reach a more beneficial place, he was able to process information and experiences and find ways to navigate his world more successfully.

In contrast, sometimes I use CST for addressing structural issues. Charlie was an eight-year-old boy with a history of significant speech and language delays. He had been in therapy for three years and had made amazing progress, and he was doing very well in school. The only thing that stood between him and graduation from speech therapy was a difficulty with the production of /r/. The distortion that he exhibited made his speech sound immature and was a source of discomfort for him. After using all the traditional approaches to working on the sound, we decided to try some CST. What I discovered through my assessment was that he had some compression in the muscles in his mouth, including his tongue, the tissues that make up the floor of the mouth, and in his jaw. Using CST to release these tensions and balance the soft tissues gave him the ability to gain motor control of the /r/ sound. We then returned to traditional SLP methods and worked on producing the sound in words, sentences, and conversation. A few months later, he was able to graduate. He is now an active and social middle school student who is doing well.

In my experience, working with children using these approaches often helps the parents as well. Sometimes children sleep or eat better following a treatment, and they seem happier, more relaxed, and more present. In recent years, I have also had some very rewarding experiences working with parents directly using these treatments. Self-care is important for parents, and both of these treatments provide both direct and indirect results that can be helpful. It should be noted that these treatments are not covered by health care plans, and not many SLPs provide them. However, you can find a qualified provider whose primary training is in another discipline and have them work with your SLP as needed. If you wish to search for a qualified CST practitioner, you can go to www.upledger.com and click on Find a Practitioner.

This chapter has covered a lot of information about your journey as a parent, and as a person. We discussed the skills and traits that seem to be present in those parents who feel and act the most effectively as advocates and parents. We also discussed the ways in which being a parent of a child with communication and developmental challenges means that you can and must act as the leader of the team working with your child. Using all of your skills and learning to trust your intuition will guide you through all the decisions that you must make over time for your child. We also discussed the use of two particular alternative treatments that I have found helpful in my practice. Hopefully, this information will provide you with some critical guidance for your own development and with hope for what is possible with effort and with persistence.

# 9

# BRINGING IT ALL TOGETHER

## Looking Ahead

As we reach the end of this book, it is a good time to look back and reflect on what we have learned so far and to think about the challenges that lie ahead. I have walked this path with many families and would like to share some final thoughts with you.

The first is that, in most cases, things get better over time. Even for children with moderate speech and language issues, things stabilize. Progress is made. Gradually, you as the parent become aware of your own strength, and that of your family. Perhaps your family becomes closer, or you and your spouse appreciate each other in a new way. Additionally, you may realize that you no longer dread the annual Individualized Education Plan (IEP) meeting because you are confident in your ability to advocate for your child and to work with his teachers and therapists to make things right.

Even the most medically involved child with communication issues can grow up and become who he is meant to be. His personality emerges, and you begin to see his potential for learning, for joy, for connection. And the child with more mild involvement, the "late talker," blossoms and eventually does not need services any more. It is easy to get caught up in the day-to-day struggles of life, or what I call the "mouse view." Mice see things up close, tiny details, . . . but they lack, cannot see, or appreciate the bigger picture.

I often speak with parents about the importance of making time to step into "eagle view" periodically. The eagle sees things from a higher perspective and is able to see the beauty and design of the whole. She may not perceive every fine detail, but she can take in the whole picture. For you as a parent, this means taking time every six months, or at least annually, to check in and review how things are going and how you are feeling about your child's progress. This may be separate from your annual or semiannual meeting where professionals give you *their* opinions about what has changed or failed to progress.

This process is for you. It is a reflection on your journey for yourself and for your child. Ask yourself some of these questions, and allow the answers to come to you:

- What can he do today that he could not do six or twelve months ago? What has that meant for him and for our family?
- What am I looking forward to next?
- What was I worried about six or twelve months ago? Am I still worried, or has that issue resolved?
- How have I been a good advocate and support for my child?
- What am I most grateful for in the past six months or year?
- Is there anything that needs to be addressed with someone on my child's team?
- What are my goals for my child now?
- What have I learned about my child in the past six months?
- Is there anyone I should thank for doing good work with my child?
- What do I want to work on for myself in the next six months?
- What will I need help with on my own journey?

These reviews are also a good time to touch base with your child's team about your concerns *and your celebrations*. Being a therapist or educator can be a tough job sometimes, and many of us give everything we have to our work. We often hear from families when they are upset or frustrated about something. However, it always touches my heart and makes me feel wonderful when a family shares a tender celebration with me. Don't be shy about celebrating your child's milestones and special moments.

## LOOKING AHEAD

For some children, speech therapy is only needed for a short time, and then it will be part of his or her history. She catches up and meets her therapy goals and then goes on to attend school with no support services needed. For other children, services will be needed for a longer time, perhaps into the school years. And a small subset of children, because of their diagnosis, may be looking at a lifetime of education plans, transition plans, and support needs. Regardless of your particular situation, looking ahead and being prepared for the next stage is important.

Children who need only short-term services generally have a positive outlook moving forward. However, the history of delay does place them at risk for later difficulties with language and reading development. In my experience, a small percentage of late talkers will end up needing some additional SLP support later on. Typically, this happens either in kindergarten as reading is being introduced, or around second grade, when the language demands in the classroom intensify. What is most important is to respond to any concerns as soon as they come up. If you or a teacher identify a problem, ask for an evaluation. Taking a deeper look at things immediately will reveal whether further services are needed, or perhaps just some strategies in the classroom. Better to be safe than sorry.

In fact, by the time a late talker gets to kindergarten, it may not even seem necessary to tell the kindergarten staff about your child's history with speech and language services. After all, it was completed years ago, and your child seems fine now. However, the course of language development is extensive and complex. If your child had a problem early on, it is quite possible that something could come up as he moves into later stages of development. If something is identified, getting help as quickly as possible will hopefully prevent any significant issues with learning academic content or with the development of frustration and low self-esteem.

Children with more significant impairments will likely continue the services they had through the schools in early childhood. You will continue to partner with your child's team to set appropriate goals and to monitor her progress within the classroom. As your child gets older, some new issues may come up that can require some careful consideration, such as:

*Educational placement*: What type of classroom is best for your child? How many students should be in the class? How many staff members? Does your child need a one-to-one aide? How similar are the students in the class? Will there be opportunities to interact with typical peers? Is your child making progress in a public school, or do they need a different kind of program?

*Therapy-life balance*: As children get older, they may receive some support services within the classroom, in the larger group. This may be beneficial because it means she is not missing classroom time for services, but she may lose the one-to-one or small-group attention she needs. However, being pulled out for services means she is missing something in the classroom. Perhaps she is missing math to work with the occupational therapist (OT), or reading to be with the SLP. Missing such classroom content means she will have to work harder to make up the missing lessons, with its resulting impact on homework. In addition, there is a social price to pay with being pulled out of the classroom while peers are watching. Some teams try to mitigate this by using "specials" time, such as art, library, or music or even recess as therapy time. While this may address the problem of missing academics, you may be asking the child to give up the one part of school where she feels best, or the one place where she can shine. You may have to work diligently with the team to determine the best solution for your child. Sometimes the best option is to shift the focus of your child's school supports and to use more outpatient treatment.

Another issue that comes up often for children with longer-term needs is *therapy burnout*. As he gets older, a child develops his own interests and wants to spend time pursuing those activities. It might be music lessons or sports, but making time for these activities can be hard when he is attending several therapy sessions a week. Sometimes you need to evaluate the bigger picture: Would your child be better served by having a break for a sports season to spend some time with peers? Doing something physical that he is interested in? Even though I believe in the power of consistent SLP services, especially when there are ongoing needs, I also have seen the impact that burnout can have on a child. He spends all his free time doing homework and attending therapy and has very little time for play dates or normal kid time. If he is not given the opportunity to have a break, he may stop participating in treatment, anyway. He may become unmotivated and detached and stop doing homework. Progress will slow down.

If you find yourself in this situation, think carefully about what would support your child right now. If his needs are long term, would it hurt to take a six-week break for the season? The same goes for summer. Having more unstructured time without the demands of school can be an opportunity to target therapy goals more intensively, but perhaps a summer where you can do things with your family, on your own schedule, would give everyone a break. Remember that language is happening everywhere, all the time. You can make any activity that you do into a language task; perhaps your SLP can even help you design some activities ahead of time that would help build your child's skills while they are learning about history or helping organize for the family trip to the beach.

*Working harder and staying behind*: In contrast to the above scenario, sometimes a child with more moderate language issues begins to experience a widening gap in academics or in his language scores compared to his peers. This means that although he is working hard in therapy, his skills are not progressing on pace with the expectations he is up against. It is at this point that you need to take stock of what you are doing and make some decisions. Will you intensify your therapy? Change your goals to focus more on compensatory strategies? As your child gets older, he should be more involved in the process. What are his goals? What would he like to work on? What is the big-picture focus moving forward?

It is also important to work with your child and your child's team to determine whether an academic college preparatory path is the right one for your child. If it seems as though it is not a good match, you may want to explore other options, such as a vocational or technical school. Some children who are not good with academics have strong aptitudes for a trade or other career path that taps into other kinds of intelligence. The long-term impact of frustration and failure can take a toll on your child, while helping him to see other possibilities may open his heart and mind to a path where he can work and have a full life doing something he enjoys.

As you move through your journey as a special needs parent, new challenges will arise. You may feel renewed grief when an important milestone passes your child by, or when a younger sibling masters a skill your older child struggled for years to learn. You may also feel anger when your child struggles to make friends. But you may also feel joy at his every accomplishment, or how polite and loving he is. As in the early part of your journey, it is important to honor your feelings as they are. Check in with yourself and determine what your needs are, and take steps to meet them.

If at any point, you feel that you are in need of support, reach out. Don't be afraid to ask for help, whether it be from your child's SLP around your child's needs, or for yourself from a counselor or support group. Living the life of a special needs parent has many gifts and many challenges. Your needs will change over the years, so you may need different kinds of support at different points in time. Know that taking care of yourself will always benefit your child and family since you are the emotional center of the family.

Bring your mind back to the earlier chapter of the book where we discussed the skills and traits that are often seen in parents who seem to be the most effective and focused and confident in managing all of their child's needs. Which ones did you identify as goals for yourself? Do you recall how you felt when you first heard your child's diagnosis? Take a gentle look at yourself now. How many of those skills are now completely within your personality? Has another parent even commented on how well you seem to handle things? Make sure to recognize your growth and evolution as much as your child's. If it had not been for your child's difficulties, you would not be who you are today. And, your child would not be who she is today without your clear heart, sharp mind, and trusted instincts.

# 10

# LESSONS I HAVE LEARNED

In over twenty years of clinical practice, I have continued to grow and expand my understanding and knowledge related to my professional identity. Aside from the fact that there are requirements for continuing education on the national and state level, speech language pathology is a field that is growing and changing all the time. Keeping up with the latest information and preferred practice patterns is both necessary and ethical. However, many of the most important and profound lessons that I have learned over the years have come from the children and families that I have had the honor to work with. This chapter is a thank-you note to all of those who have made me who I am as a clinician; I am proud to share these lessons with you now. These "golden nuggets" represent many of the untold and unwritten aspects of being a strong, compassionate, and helpful speech language pathologist.

## LESSON NUMBER ONE

*Relationships are the key to success.* This is such an important point that I have chosen to share it as the first thing I want you to know. Not only is a bond or relationship the key to unlocking communication in the earliest stages, it actually underlies successful therapeutic relationships in every setting and with every child, regardless of age, diagnosis, or ability. Having solid clinical skills, excellent training, and a desire to help can only take you so far. The chemistry that exists between an SLP and a child (and by extension the family) can be a powerful force for progress, or it can be the factor that derails the whole process. Some of my most profound experiences came in the days of my residency, when my clinical knowledge and experience were mere shadows of what they are today. And even as a seasoned clinician, there have been children and families who were not a right fit for me. Tuning in to how your child relates to the SLP you are working with can sometimes give you more information than the diplomas on the wall. Meeting your child where he is, and creatively tapping into his interests and helping him become a successful communicator, is based in large part on how your child feels when he is with the SLP. As we know, a child under stress is not going to learn as well as one that is happy, or at least relaxed. Be confident in your assessment of that relationship, and make changes if necessary. Years of experience alone do not tell you what you need to know. Does your child like going to speech sessions? Does he seem happy and excited when you pull up to the building? Does he greet the SLP and seem eager to go? Does he indicate that he had fun? How do you feel when you transition your child into a session? Remember that *you know what you know.* Likewise, do you feel comfortable asking questions? Do you understand what your child is working on and why? Do you have an easy, warm relationship with the SLP?

## LESSON NUMBER TWO

*Everything is a conversation.* This lesson is a corollary to the first. I began to understand this lesson when I worked in the neonatal intensive care unit (NICU) with premature infants and their families. Obviously, premature infants cannot speak, but they do communicate. They use a wide variety of nonverbal signals, such as skin color, eye gaze, body tone, and even sucking their thumb to tell you everything you need to know about how they are feeling in the moment. My job as an SLP was to teach parents to see what was already there, to tune in to these subtle signals, and to respond in ways that the baby could handle. Likewise, with toddlers who fail to develop their communication skills, my job is to tune in to the ways that they *are already* trying to communicate and to help parents connect the dots and see the messages. Once you understand the signals your child uses, you can begin to connect more meaningfully with him. As children grow and their skills progress, this lesson still applies. Any time we offer a new treatment program, technique, or activity, we have to look at how the child is responding and adapt ourselves, if necessary, in order to facilitate learning. Expressing subtle and abstract emotions or concepts can remain challenging for children with speech and language disorders for years; we must work hard to read him and modify the supports, our expectations, or the context as needed. In the NICU, parents learn to "ask the baby." In later years, it is appropriate to ask, "How is my child receiving this? Is there anything I need to change to help him get it?"

## LESSON NUMBER THREE

*Every child has an "X factor."* Some might call it *spirit*, or *personality*, or *soul*. Every child has a force inside of her that cannot be accounted for by tests, diagnoses, or even the experience and wisdom of doctors or teachers or therapists. While there may be some information available to you about what to expect in the long term, it is important to know that children sometimes far surpass what is predicted in the days after birth. I will never forget Sally, a little girl I worked with on both communication and feeding skills. She had been born at twenty-five weeks, almost four months early, and she had a challenging medical course with many complications. Her parents were told that she might never walk or talk or feed herself, and to keep their expectations low for what she might be able to do. They did not know Sally. Although her work in treatment was hard, Sally always had an amazing spirit. Her parents were so proud on the day they put her down in the hallway of the doctor's office and she *ran* down the hall yelling "helloooooooooooo" to the nurse. When it seems like things are going rough, and your enthusiasm and strength are fading, remember Sally. Tune in to your own special child and connect with that light inside of her. Foster it and be grateful for it. And when doctors or other professionals tell you what *"will* be," know that they don't always *know what you know.* They are giving you the benefit of their experience, or the typical course they may have seen before. Let your child show you her way.

## LESSON NUMBER FOUR

*Tests don't tell the whole story.* This lesson goes hand in hand with Lesson Three. Professionals such as SLPs are tasked with the job of quantifying (assigning a number or score) your child's difficulties, which is not always easy. Some children have significant difficulty with participating in such high-demand activities as tests, and some children are simply not able to complete anything so out of context as performing on a test. Even for older children, our formal tests require a child to demonstrate skills in the absence of any cues or supports because to provide those supports invalidates the scores. Yet every six months or year, you may be presented with the latest round of numbers that are meant to describe your child, and each time it may trigger negative emotions for you. For many kinds of communication disorders, there are very few tests that can accurately capture the full picture of your child's strengths and needs. This is why SLPs frequently use non–standardized tests to gather other useful information about how your child is currently functioning so that a good treatment plan can be developed. When you are faced with the prospect of hearing about scores, pause and take a breath. Look at the bigger picture. Do the scores show that change has occurred since the last evaluation? What about test-taking behavior, like being able to stay on task or showing less anxiety? Ask questions about how well your child is *communicating* now, in addition to the scores. What does the testing truly tell about your child and how she is learning and interacting?

## LESSON NUMBER FIVE

*A diagnosis is often just a label.* For some parents, getting a diagnosis and having a *name* for a child's difficulties is important. Perhaps it gives you a place to begin reading to understand more about your child's challenges. Or maybe having a particular diagnosis gives you access to services and resources you would otherwise be unable to receive. For other parents, a diagnosis feels like a final statement, a proclamation about who your child can be or what he can achieve. The danger of this is that you begin to shape your expectations and gear your thoughts toward whatever the conventional wisdom says about that diagnosis.

Remember that tests don't tell us everything and that every child has an "X factor." You should know that in many instances, the kind of supports used by SLPs, targeted specifically for your child's unique issues, drive the development of your child's plan, regardless of the diagnosis. Generally speaking, I would not teach vocabulary differently to a child with a language delay from one with persistent ear infections. The methodology is the same, but the supports, cues, and strategies I use may be different. When moving through your process, keep this in mind when looking for a diagnosis. Often, it is really just a label—all the critical information for successful intervention is within your child.

## LESSON NUMBER SIX

*Conventional wisdom changes.* As we come to understand more about the human brain, communication, and the genetic basis of many disorders, clinicians are faced with the challenge of evaluating new information in light of prior knowledge and experience. The profession of speech language pathology is young by many standards, and significant new discoveries are made all the time through both traditional scientific and clinical research. It is important to keep an open mind about new information and to talk with your SLP about new ideas and opportunities. However, with each new understanding comes a period of adjustment and integration. There is no need to throw out methods that are working for your child in favor of something new. And technology is not the answer to every problem. Technology has an important role to play, but it cannot replace the power of person-to-person communication. Recall that things often happen in cycles, and that there is always time to try new approaches and to see how your child responds. No treatment works for everyone, nor is everything new necessarily better. When you hear about a new treatment program or technique, talk about it with your SLP and determine together if it might be appropriate for your child.

## LESSON NUMBER SEVEN

*Children must be motivated in order to make progress.* Every parent has had the experience of using the promise of a reward to compel a child to do something he does not want to do. This can be a time-consuming and ineffective process for promoting true changes in behavior. For the SLP working with your child, there usually has to be a combination of internal and external dedication and effort for true progress to be made. For most children who have difficulty learning to communicate, speech therapy involves nothing short of having a laser-like focus on the task that is hardest for him in life. Even as adults, we try to avoid things that are challenging and want to spend our energy where it is easy to see results. In younger children, this means using toys and activities that they prefer, especially when targeting skills that are difficult. A good SLP should be able to target a variety of goals no matter what the toy is, so there is no reason to constantly push toward activities and games that don't capture his interest. For older children, this might mean using favorite topics, such as superheroes or trains, as the context for language activities. If he is interested, he has the potential to learn.

## LESSON NUMBER EIGHT

*Stressed systems don't strengthen.* This was discussed in an earlier chapter, but it is a lesson frequently reinforced when you spend time working with children. Children who feel safe and who are calmer and happier are more likely to learn and retain new information. Have you ever tried taking a class or learning a new skill, something that scares you or causes a lot of anxiety about doing well? Those stressors literally cause biochemical changes in your brain and body that can inhibit your ability to listen and learn.[1] In these moments, you become physically prepared to flee with the activation of the survival parts of your brain. As noted above, tune in to how your child approaches things that are challenging for her. What supports can you offer to help minimize her stress? Likewise, your SLP should be thinking about this and offering practical strategies as well.

## LESSON NUMBER NINE

*Behaviors are not always what they seem.* It is true that behavior is *always* communication, but the first interpretation may not always the accurate one. Not long ago, I was working with David and his mother in a session. David is a two-year-old boy with a genetic syndrome that causes significant speech and language delays. David also has some sensory-processing challenges, and although he works hard, he gets frustrated and overwhelmed at times. Mom asked me one day if it was normal or okay that David liked to lie on the floor and watch objects up close. Although we know that David is not on the autism spectrum, another therapist had told mom that this was "stimming" behavior (self-stimulatory behavior often associated with autism) and that she should work to discourage and, hopefully, eliminate it. As we talked about this behavior, David seized the opportunity to engage in his "looking" while the spotlight was off him. The more we talked about it, the more it became clear that David was *using* this behavior to soothe himself, to calm his nervous system, and in fact to try to activate his visual system, which was impaired. He was easily redirected from the behavior and usually stopped on his own when he met the need that caused this particular behavior. That day, we discovered that David had stumbled upon his own best sensory strategy and that there was no need to try to change it. While not every behavior is acceptable or socially appropriate, it is important to look deeper at it, especially for children who don't communicate easily or well. We all have strategies that we use to calm ourselves or to promote well-being when we feel down or off. Look at the behavior and ask yourself questions, such as, When does this behavior show up? How intense is it? How easily can it be interrupted or redirected? What purpose is it serving? Then work with your SLP to determine whether the behavior needs to be changed or just witnessed.

## LESSON NUMBER TEN

*Children need breaks.* Working on building speech and language skills or overcoming a developmental challenge is a monumental challenge by any standard. This lesson reminds us that we need to be aware of how much cognitive and sometimes physical effort is required in therapy.

And, as parents and therapists, we need to appreciate the way that the brain works when learning something new. There is usually a period of intense input and practice, followed by a period of integration. In terms of day-to-day considerations, this may mean allowing your child to have some down time after therapy or when she seems to be overwhelmed. It may also mean taking periodic breaks from treatment when your child seems burned out and less able to focus and make progress. No one goes full force all the time; we need to have a balance in time for our brain to work and then to rest. Look carefully at your weekly schedule, and be sure that you are not wasting time, money, or effort pushing so hard at your goals that your child's nervous system has shut down in the process. In addition, many families of children with challenges feel they should skip family outings and vacations to maintain consistency and routine. While this may be important at certain points in your child's development, it is also often the case that getting out of your routine and spending some unstructured time together can be a catalyst for the integration of learned communication skills mentioned above. Know that it is okay to let off the gas pedal sometimes.

## LESSON NUMBER ELEVEN

*Children don't always make progress in a linear way.* When a child begins therapy, it is usually relatively easy to determine his learning style and how he likes to take in new information. What may not be as easy to see right away is the overall pattern of his learning. If you take a "typical" nervous system, and task it with learning a new skill, chances are you would see a relatively slow but steady upward arc of improved ability. Practice makes perfect, and the more practice, the more that speed, accuracy, and precision increases. This is not always the case for children with speech and language issues. Because the nervous system may not be typical, extra support to learn new skills may be required. Often, these children tend to exhibit more of a "stair-step" pattern of progress. In practical terms, this means that he may make big leaps and then integrate for some length of time, when he can practice and refine the new skill. Often, before he makes a leap or acquires some new skill, his behavior overall may seem to regress. It can be mystifying to suddenly see things that had come along get lost, and children can become irritable and more frustrated than usual. Then suddenly, everything evens out. When you become aware that your child exhibits this pattern, observing the "falling apart" can actually lead to "happy anticipation" of what is coming next!

On a related note, children who are working hard to master one skill sometimes seem to lose skills in other areas. This is because the developing brain only has so much cognitive reserve, and when there is intense focus in one area, such as learning to walk, everything else can get deemphasized. Usually, once the new skill is in place, the others will come back naturally. This is often seen in children who are learning to communicate as well. Communication progress suddenly seems to slow down when the motor system takes over. Likewise, if he is working hard on talking, he may need more support around balance and coordination.

## LESSON NUMBER TWELVE

*It is all about the art of redirection.* Helping children, especially toddlers, navigate successfully through the day can be a tall order. When you add communication or developmental delays into that equation, it can seem overwhelming. And when you further add the "terrible twos," it can seem nearly impossible to get out the door. In working with children for so many years, it has become clear to me that how you talk about tasks and how you present demands make a big difference. Children are always on the lookout for anything that feels like a demand and may sometimes seem to resist on principle. The job of the adult is to make the demand seem like something they cannot resist doing. One area where this often shows up is cleanup time. If a child is asked to put toys away, she will often say "no" and refuse to comply. However, when asked to drive the cars into the garage, or to jump the little people into a box, she will usually cooperate, because of the way the task was presented. Although there are certainly times when you must present a clear demand to your child, you will be more successful and feel less frustrated if you can find ways to tap into creativity and fun while doing it. This approach also makes those clear demands stand out. This is related to another lesson, about *providing the illusion of control.* Children must learn to assert themselves and to express their wants and needs in the first few years of life. It may often seem that his wants and needs are in direct opposition to yours, and he completely disregards the time constraints you may be up against. It is at these times when you have to choose between providing a choice to your child or setting a firm limit. In the case of offering choices, be sure that you are giving two options that are acceptable to you. "Do you want your left shoe or your right?" may seem like a silly choice, but giving that illusion of control is sometimes all you need to break a stalemate. In the event that you need to set a firm limit, be sure that your language matches your message. If there is no time left to play, and it is time to get dressed, avoid asking your child, "Do you want to get dressed now?" If you pose the question that way, you have only a fifty-fifty chance that the answer will be "yes." Far more likely is that you will hear "no," and he will go back to playing. When you use the language, "Time to get dressed," you communicate the unilateral nature of your decision and can begin to move along.

## LESSON NUMBER THIRTEEN

*Sleep, water, and good nutrition are critical to the health and success of both you and your child.* Everyone knows the value of a good night's sleep or the chaos that can be created when your child's nap schedule is thrown off. What you may not realize is how important sleep is to your physical and mental health. When you or your child are deprived of good quality sleep, it can cause poor immunity and mood disorders, and it can make you more susceptible to accidents.[2] If your child is not sleeping well, work with your doctor to find out *why.* Is there something in your child's room that causes her to remain overstimulated? Is there a medical problem, such as sleep apnea, that is keeping her from reaching a deep sleep? If you are the one experiencing the sleep challenge, consult with your physician to find out why. Is your thyroid in a state of dysfunction? Are you worrying about your child or other challenges and can't turn off your brain? What is most important is that you work to address the root causes and not just the symptoms. The same is true for your child. When your child is able to have good sleep, this provides the brain with essential rest and the ability to take on the challenges of tomorrow. In the same way, the importance of being hydrated and eating well cannot be overemphasized. Just as the body needs adequate sleep to function well, being dehydrated can affect your entire body, as well as your endurance. Poor hydration can also cause headaches and digestive problems.[3] For you and your child, being hydrated is literally feeding the brain. Our bodies are made up of 75 percent water, and it is closer to 90 percent for the brain.[4] Ask your pediatrician how much water your child should have, and strive to limit sugary drinks like juice and soda during the day. Modeling good habits is important, too. Finally, the brain is also fed by good nutrition. Many parents today are incorporating more organic and whole foods into their child's daily routine. This should be encouraged. But for every mom who makes her own organic foods, there are others who are struggling to feed picky eaters who only want and accept foods that have a lot of sugar, salt, and fat. If your child restricts their eating to these kinds of foods, seek help from your SLP. If your clinician does not treat feeding issues, she may be able to refer you to someone in your area who does.

## LESSON NUMBER FOURTEEN

SLPs can only help you based the information they have been given. Even the most skilled SLP cannot infer what is happening in your home and in your life unless they are working with you in that context. It is up to you to fill in the gaps that make the bigger picture for us, so that we can tailor treatment and expectations for home practice in ways that feel responsive and possible for you. If you are having a bad day, or a rough month, even if it is about something completely outside of the realm of speech therapy, allow yourself to share that with your therapist. The SLP may be able to provide you with empathetic listening, support, ideas, or resources that may help you. If nothing else, you can be seen and heard, as you are, in the moment. The value of that alone can be worth a lot, and it will foster the relationship between the two of you. In addition, it will prevent the SLP from making assumptions about your feelings regarding therapy or the value you place on it in your child's life.

## LESSON NUMBER FIFTEEN

*Everyone changes.* This point is being included as a reminder to you as the parent that SLPs are people, too, and we have strengths and weaknesses just like anyone else. There may be times when your SLP is facing some challenging circumstances of her own, and your understanding and patience is invaluable. This also means that there are times when a child may simply stop making progress for a time, either due to their condition, or their stage of development. In most situations, this is no one's fault. If you have tried modifying things with no success, sometimes you need to end the relationship with your SLP. Conversely, sometimes your SLP may determine that you have reached the end of your work together and that it is time to move on. It is important to determine whether the SLP is saying that your child is not likely to make further progress or if you just need a change in clinician. Relationships grow, they change, and sometimes they end. Bless them for what they have meant to you, and move on.

Every family that I have worked with has taught me something. I have shared many of those lessons with you here. When you are working with your SLP, know that she is learning as much from you as you are from her. I know that the children I have worked with stay with me long after they leave my practice and that they leave an imprint on my heart. These special children have shaped my development as a clinician, and they have taught me a lot about what it means to be human and to share the power of communication.

# APPENDIX A

## Speech Sound Development

Please note that there is a wide range of variability in when children master speech sounds. Each sound typically emerges in a child's speech over time, usually appearing at the beginning or end of words first, followed by the middle position. For example, a child who is learning to say the /b/ sound might learn to say it in "ball" and then "tub" before "cubby."

As children are learning sounds, they may be inconsistent in their ability to make the sound, or make mistakes based on the sounds around that particular target. In addition, each sound is easier to make in simple words than in *multisyllable* words. Using the example with /b/ above, it is much easier to say, "ball" than "basketball." Consider the list below a guideline, a place to begin a dialogue with your child's speech language pathologist (SLP). Keep in mind that there are regional and *dialectal* variations to consider as well. In the area where I live in Massachusetts, many children exhibit a Boston accent, which radically changes their production of the /r/ sound. That is taken into consideration when determining whether a particular pattern in a child's speech is indicative of a disorder or merely an acceptable part of the local tongue.

For most children, sounds are mastered at or around the ages shown in table A.1.

**Table A.1 Age of Mastery for Consonant Sounds**

| Age in Years | Sounds Typically Mastered at This Age |
|---|---|
| Two years | /p/, /b/, /m/, /n/, /w/, /h/ are emerging |
| Three years | /p/, /b/, /m/, /n/, /w/, /h/ are mastered; /b/ is emerging |
| Four years . | /b/, /k/, /g/, /d/, /f/, /y/ ("yuck"); /t/ and /ng/ ("sing") are emerging |
| Five years | /r/, /l/, /s/, /ch/, /sh/, /z/, /j/ ("jump") and /v/ are emerging |
| Six years | /t/, /ng/, /r/,* /l/ are mastered; /th/ and /zh/ ("treasure") are emerging |
| Seven years | /ch/, /sh/, /j/ mastered |
| Eight years | /s/, /z/, /v/, /th/, /zh/ mastered |

*Mastery of /r/ can take up to eight years, and there is dialectal variation as well. In children with a strong Boston accent, it may never be mastered at the end of words.

*Source:* Data taken from E. Sander, "When Are Speech Sounds Learned?" *Journal of Speech and Hearing Disorders.* 37, no.1 (1972): 55–63.

# APPENDIX B

## Channeling Your Emotions

Feel free to use this exercise whenever you need to work out some complicated feelings or when you just want to dig a bit deeper into what you are feeling.

First, find a time when you can be quiet and without distractions for five to ten minutes. If you are using your phone for quiet and peaceful music, disable your phone so that you will not be disturbed.

Second, find a comfortable position and close your eyes. Take a few deep breaths and center yourself. You can expect that when you try to quiet your mind, your thoughts may run wild, and you may feel as if your mind is spinning in circles. Focus on your breathing. Just listen to the sound of your breath as it travels in and out, and let whatever thoughts come up drift away.

When you are ready, tune in to the emotion that you are seeking to connect with and understand. Let it "bubble up" and allow yourself to feel it completely, without judgment. Whatever this feeling is, it can move through you if you allow it. Let that emotion build and change. You may feel physical symptoms, such as flushing, tightness in your gut or chest, rapid pulse, or others. This is normal. Observe the process as if you are watching yourself; focus on your breathing, and stay present for yourself in the moment.

After about ninety seconds, or maybe a bit longer, you will feel the emotion begin to fade and find yourself feeling more "in control." Stay present with yourself as you move through this process. Once you feel as though the emotion has subsided, take a few more deep breaths and bring yourself back to the room where you are. Slowly open your eyes and feel your fingers and toes; stretch and move a bit. When you are ready, answer the following questions. Remember that this is for you, and your eyes only, unless you choose to share it.

1. What was the emotion that came up for you?
2. How did it "show up" in your physical body?
3. How did it change over the course of the few moments when you allowed yourself to feel it fully?
4. What did your experience of this emotion teach you or show you? Do you need to seek some emotional support? Do you have a need that is not being met?
5. What have you now opened up by allowing yourself to fully feel this emotion? Do you now see actions that need to be taken? Do you feel cared for? Do you just feel relief?
6. What will you do differently now?

# RESOURCES

You may wish to consult some of these organizations and agencies for more information about the topics discussed in this book. This list is not meant to be exhaustive, but to provide you with a place to begin looking more deeply into a topic.

The American Academy of Audiology—www.howsyourhearing.org
Information about hearing loss and related topics in adults and children. Also has a searchable database to find an audiologist near you.

The American Speech Language Hearing Association—www.asha.org
ASHA is the professional credentialing organization for speech language pathology. Their website portal provides information written for the general public on topics related to communication disorders. There is also a portal, Find a Practitioner, if you wish to search for certified professionals in your area.

The Autism Society of America—www.autism-society.org
The Autism Society is a grassroots organization dedicated to spreading awareness about autism, advocating for the needs of those with autism, and supporting education and research.

The Federation for Children with Special Needs—www.fcsn.org
The Federation for Children is an organization based in Boston, Massachusetts. They offer parent support around issues related to educational

advocacy. FCSN also offers training in advocacy and referrals to qualified trained advocates who can help you with your child's specific educational program.

The Hanen Centre—www.hanen.org
The Hanen Centre is a nonprofit charitable organization that offers education and educational products specifically aimed at supporting parents in becoming language facilitators for young children.

Individuals with Disabilities Education Act—http://idea.ed.gov
This website is described as a "one-stop shop" for all kinds of information related to special education, including your rights, help in understanding the provisions of special education law, and the various programs outlined within the law.

International Center for Reiki Training—www.reiki.org
The ICRT offers an expansive library of articles related to the history, development, and use of Reiki in the United States. ICRT also houses articles and information on past and current research about the use of Reiki with a variety of medical conditions, as well as information about training and how to find a practitioner in your area.

Learning Disabilities Online—www.ldonline.org
LD Online is the largest online resource for information related to learning disabilities.

The Mighty—www.facebook.com/themightysite
The Mighty is a Facebook-based forum that posts articles and stories about a wide range of disabilities, many of them written by parents of children with special needs. Part education and part support, but nearly always a source of inspiration.

The National Institute for Deafness and Communication Disorders—www.nidcd.hin.gov
The NIDCD conducts research in, and provides information and education on, a wide range of topics related to disorders of human communication. Easy-to-search database.

Sign2Me—www.sign2me.com
Another leading online resource for accessing high-quality educational products designed to teach ASL signs to young children. Also offers educator training and Find A Class near you.

Signing Times—www.signingtime.com
Online store for educational resources, DVDs, and other products designed to teach American Sign Language (ASL) to young children.

Stop Bullying—www.stopbullying.gov
Provides information and resources about bullying, including, state by state, laws and regulations.

The Stuttering Foundation of America—www.stutteringhelp.org
The Stuttering Foundation is a nonprofit organization dedicated to the support of people who stutter. The site offers many educational products, DVDs, posters, and other materials. This site also offers a referral directory for finding a practitioner near you.

Talking with Children—www.talkingwithchildren.com
A website designed by speech language pathologist, Dr. Rae Banigan, CCC-SLP. Her site offers specific step-by-step lessons on how to facilitate language development in young children.

The Upledger Institute—www.upledger.com
The Upledger Institute provides information and education about craniosacral therapy and related therapies. This is the primary source of training for Upledger-trained practitioners. Also connects with a referral database for finding a practitioner near you.

Wrightslaw—www.wrightslaw.com
The largest online resource for information about special education law and advocacy.

# NOTES

## 1. WELCOME TO THE JOURNEY

1.  Emily Perl Kingsley, "Welcome to Holland," www.our-kids.org, 1987; www.our-kids.org/Archives/Holland.html.

2.  National Institute on Deafness and Other Communication Disorders (NIDCD), www.nidcd.nih.gov/health/stats/vsl/Pages/stats.aspx.

3.  National Institute of Mental Health (NIMH), www.nimh.nih.gov/health/topics/autism-spectrum-disorders-asd/index.shtml.

4.  NIDCD, www.nidcd.nih.gov/health/statistics/vsl/Pages/Comm-disorders.aspx.

5.  Myers Briggs Foundation, www.myersbriggs.org/my-mbti-personality-type/mbti-basics.

6.  Personalitypathways.com, www.personalitypathways.com.

7.  Ball State University website, cms.bsu.edu/about/administrative-offices/careercenter.

8.  John E. Upledger and Jon Vredevoogd, *Craniosacral Therapy.* (Seattle: Eastland Press, 1983.)

9.  John E. Upledger, *Pediatrics 2 Study Guide.* (Florida: UI Publishing. Revised 2009.)

10.  John E. Upledger, *CST 1 Study Guide*, rev. ed. (Florida: UI Publishing, 2006.)

11.  Dustin Fink, "Concussion: After Injury Care," *Concussion* (blog). March 5, 2012.

12.  Tad Wanveer, "Autism Spectrum Disorders: How CST Can Help," *Massage Today* 7 (2007): 1–4.

13.  www.asha.org/members/ebp/Introduction-to-Evidence-Based-Practice.

14.  . "Listening to the Body: Understanding the Language of Stress Related Symptoms," May 2012 course materials


## 2. ALPHABET SOUP AND SEEING YOUR CHILD IN CONTEXT


1.  American Speech Language Hearing Association. *National Outcomes Measurement System: Pre-K Speech Language Pathology Training Manual Functional Communication Measures* (Rockville, MD: ASHA, 2003.)

2.  Kristin R. Stickler, *Guide to Analysis of Language Transcripts* (Eau Claire, WI: Thinking Publications, 1987.)


## 3. COMMUNICATION DEVELOPMENT


1.  Jeri L Miller, "Pediatrics Primer! From Embryo-to-Infant: Developmental Biology of Feeding-Swallowing-Respiratory Systems." Paper presented at the annual ASHA Convention (Philadephia, PA, November 2004).

2.  Psychology.about.com, www.psychology.about.com/od/cognitivepsychology/a/left-brain-right-brain.htm.

3.  A. Jean Ayres, *Sensory Integration and the Child* (Los Angeles: Western Psychological Services, 1979.)

4.  Mary Sue Williams and Shelly Shellenberger, *How Does Your Engine Run? Leader's Guide to the Alert Program for Self-Regulation* (Albuquerque, NM: Therapy Works, 1996.)


## 4. ASSESSMENT OF SPEECH AND LANGUAGE DISORDERS


1.  Dale Purves et al., eds., *Neuroscience*, 5th ed. (Sunderland, MA: Sinauer Associates, 2011).


## 5. AN OVERVIEW OF SPEECH SOUND DISORDERS


1.  R. Prezas and Barbara Hodson, "Phonological Cycles Remedial Approach," in *Interventions for Speech Sound Disorders in Children*, eds. (Baltimore: Brookes Publishing, 2010), 137–57.

2.  Nancy Swigert, "Dysarthria: Understanding and Assessing." Class presented by Linguisystems, Inc., November 2013.

3. Nancy Swigert, "Dysarthria: Practical Approaches to Treatment." Class presented by Linguisystems, Inc. November 2013.

4. Prezas and Hodson, "Phonological Cycles Remedial Approach."

5. Apraxia-Kids, www.apraxia-kids.org/guides/slp-start-guide/key-charac-teristics-of-cas.

6. Ibid.

7. R. Prezas, and Barbara Hodson, "Phonological Cycles Remedial Approach."

## 6. AN OVERVIEW OF LANGUAGE DISORDERS

1. NIDCD, www.nidcd.nih.gov/health/statistics/vsl/Pages/Comm-disorders.aspx.

2. Jan Pepper and Elaine Weitzman, *It Takes Two to Talk*, 3rd ed. (Toronto: Hanen Early Language Program, 2004).

3. Babysignlanguage.com, www.babysignlanguage.com/basics/research.

4. Kristine R. Stickler, *Guide to Analysis of Language Transcripts* (Eau Claire, WI: Thinking Publications, 1987).

5. Dorinne Davis, *A Parent's Guide to Middle Ear Infections.* (Hear You Are, Inc., 1994.)

6. Stopbullying.gov.

7. Autism Speaks, *www.autismspeaks.org/what-autism/treatment/applied-behavior-analysis.* Autismspeaks.org, accessed December 15, 2015.

8. James R. Laidler, "The Refrigerator Mother Hypothesis of Autism," Austim-watch.org, www.autism-watch/org/causes/rm/shtml, accessed December 1, 2015.

9. G. Steinman et al., eds., *The Cause of Autism: Concepts and Misconceptions.* (New York: Baffin Books, 2014).

10. www.nimh.nih.gov/health/topics/autism-spectrum-disorder-asd.index.shtml.

11. www.autismspeaks.org/what-autism/treatment/applied-behavior-analysis.

12. March of Dimes, www.marchofdimes.org.

13. Heidelise Als et al., "Early Experience Alters Brain Function and Structure" in *Pediatrics* 113 (April 2004): 846–57.

## 7. THE PARENT EXPERIENCE

1. Raphael Cushnir, *The One Thing Holding You Back: Unleashing the Power of Emotional Connection* (New York: HarperOne, 2008).

2. Dick Sobsey, "Marital Stability and Marital Satisfaction in Families of Children with Disabilities: Chicken or Egg?" *Developmental Disabilities Bulletin* 32 (2004): 62–83.

## 8. FINDING THE NEW NORMAL

1. The Federation for Children with Special Needs, fcsn.org.

2. Elizabeth Kubler-Ross, *On Death and Dying* (New York: Scribner, 1969).

3. Reiki.org,, www.Reiki.org.

4. Ibid.

## 10. LESSONS I HAVE LEARNED

1. John Upledger, *Pediatrics 2 Study Guide*, rev. ed. (Florida: UI Publishing, 2009).

2. WebMd, www.webmd.com/sleep-disorders/excessive.sleepiness/10/10-results-sleep-loss.

3. Nancy Hearn, "Dehydration: Effects of Water Loss in the Human Body," www.waterbenefitshealth.com/dehydration.effects.html, accessed December 5, 2015.

4. Chemistry.about.com/od/waterchemistry/f/how-much-of-your-body-is-water.htm.

# BIBLIOGRAPHY

Als, Heidelise. "Earliest Intervention for Preterm Infants in the Newborn Intensive Care Unit." In *The Effectiveness of Early Intervention*, edited by Michael J. Guralnick, 47–76. Baltimore: Brookes Publishing, 1996.

———. "Neurodevelopment and Experience: Evidence for Developmentally Supportive Care in the NICU." Paper presented at the annual ASHA Convention, Boston, MA. November 2007.

———. "A Synactive Model of Neonatal Behavioral Organization: A Framework for the Assessment of Neurobehavioral Development in the Preterm Infant and for Supporting Infants and Parents in the NICU." In *The High-Risk Neonate: Developmental Therapy Perspectives in Physical and Occupational Therapy in Pediatrics*, edited by J. K. Sweeney. New York: Hawork Press, 1986.

Als, Heidelise, F. H. Duffy, G. B. McAnulty, M. J. Rivkin, S. Vajapeyam, R. V. Mulkern, S. K. Warfield et al. "Early Experience Alters Brain Function and Structure." *Pediatrics* 113, no. 4 (2004): 846–57.American Speech Language Hearing Association. Information on evidence-based practice. www.asha.org/members/ebp/Introduction-to-Evidence-Based-Practice. Accessed December 5, 2015.

American Speech Language Hearing Association. *National Outcomes Measurement System: Pre-K Speech Language Pathology Training Manual Functional Communication Measures*. Rockville, MD: ASHA, 2003.

Apraxia-Kids. Apraxia-kids.org. Accessed December 1, 2015.

Autism Speaks. *www.autismspeaks.org/what-autism/treatment/applied-behavior-analysis*. Autismspeaks.org. Accessed December 15, 2015.

Ayres, A. Jean, and Jeff Robbins. *Sensory Integration and the Child*. Los Angeles: Western Psychological Services, 1979.

Babysignlanguage.com. *www.babysignlanguage.com/basics/research*. Accessed 11/30/15.

Ball State University website. *cms.bsu.edu/about/administrative-offices/careercenter*. Accessed November 26, 2015.

Banigan, Rae L. *A Family Centered Approach to Developing Communication: Prevention, Screening and Facilitation*. Boston: Butterworth-Heinemann, 1998.

Chemistry.about.com. *www.chemistry.about.com/od/waterchemistry/f/how-much-of-your-body-is-water.htm*. Accessed December 1, 2015.

Cloherty, John P., and Ann Stark, eds. *Manual of Neonatal Care*. 4th ed. Philadelphia: Lippincott William and Walkins, 1998.

Cushnir, Raphael. *The One Thing Holding You Back: Unleashing the Power of Emotional Connection*. New York: HarperOne, 2008.

Davis, Dorinne. *A Parent's Guide to Middle Ear Infections*. Stanhope, NJ: Hear You Are, 1994.

Dawson, Peg. "Smart but Scattered: Executive Dysfunction at Home and School." Course taken via PESI, June 16, 2015.

Dawson, Peg, and Richard Guare. *Smart but Scattered*. New York: Guilford Press, 2009.

Deal, L. V. and W. H. Haas. "Hearing and the Development of Language and Speech." *Folia Phoniatrica and Logopaedica* 48, no. 3 (1996): 111–16.

Degangi, Georgia, Cecilia Breinbauer, Jane D. Roosevelt, Stephen Forges, and Stanley Greenspan. "Prediction of Childhood Problems at Three Years in Children Experiencing Disorders of Regulation During Infancy." *Infant Mental Health Journal* 21, no. 3 (2000): 156–75.

Fink, Dustin. "Concussion: After Injury Care." The Concussion Blog. www.thecon cussionblog.com. March 5, 2012.

Hathaway, Beth. "Early Intervention Strategies for Family Centered Care." Course material. Dedham, MA, March 25, 2015.

Hearn, Nancy. "Dehydration: Effects of Water Loss in the Human Body." http://www.waterbenefitshealth.com/dehydration.effects.html. Accessed December 5, 2015.

Kingsley, Emily P. "Welcome to Holland." 1987. www.our-kids.org, 1987, www.our-kids.org/Archives/Holland.html.

Kranowitz, Carol Stock. *The Out-of-Sync Child*. New York: Berkley Publishers, 1998.

Kubler-Ross, Elizabeth. *On Death and Dying*. New York: Scribner, 1969.

Laidler, James R. "The Refrigerator Mother Hypothesis of Autism." www.autism-watch/org/causes/rm/shtml. Accessed December 1, 2015.

Lanza, Janet, and Lynn Flahive. *Guide to Communication Milestones*. Eau Claire, WI: Linguisystems, Inc. 2008.

Love, Russell J. *Childhood Motor Speech Disability*. New York: Macmillan, 1992.

Love, Russell J., and Wanda G. Webb. *Neurology for the Speech Language Pathologist*. Boston: Butterworth-Heinemann, 1996.

March of Dimes. www.marchofdimes.org. Accessed November 25, 2015.

Miller, Jeri L. "Pediatrics Primer! From Embryo-to-Infant: Developmental Biology of Feeding-Swallowing-Respiratory Systems." Paper presented at the annual ASHA Convention, Philadephia, PA. November 2004.

Moraine, Paula. "Dyslexia, ADHD and Executive Function." Course offered via PESI. May 14, 2014.

Myers Briggs Foundation. www.meyersbriggs.org/my-mbti-personalitytype/mbti-basics. Accessed December 1, 2015.

Offenbacher, Barbara L. *First Words: A Parent's Step-By-Step Guide to Helping a Child with Speech and Language Delays*. New York: Rowman and Littlefield, 2013.

Pepper, Jan and Elaine Weitzman. *It Takes Two to Talk*, 3rd ed. Ontario: Hanen Early Language Program, 2004.

Personalitypathways.com. Information about results of Myers-Briggs Test. www.personalitypathways.com. Accessed December 1, 2015.

Prezas, R., and B. Hodson. "Phonological Cycles Remedial Approach." In *Interventions for Speech Sound Disorders in Children*, edited by L. Williams, S. McLeod, and R. McCauley, 137–57. Baltimore: Brookes Publishing, 2010.

Prizant, Barry, with Tom Fields-Meyer. *Uniquely Human*. New York: Simon and Schuster, 2015.

Prizant, Barry. "Enhancing Communication and Socioemotional Competence in Young Children with Autism and Pervasive Developmental Disorders. Course Information. Boston: Emerson College, 1992.

Psychology.about.com. Information about brain dominance. www.psychology.about.com/od/cognitivepsychology/a/left-brain-right-brain.htm. Accessed December 1, 2015.

Purves, D., G. Augustine, D. Fitzpatrick, W. C. Hall, A. S. LaMantia, and Leonard E. White, eds. *Neuroscience*, 5th ed. Sunderland, MA: Sinauer Associates, 2011.

Reiki.org. Website for the International Center for Reiki Training. www.reiki.org. Accessed November 1, 2015.

Roland, Melinda and Sally Frier Dietz. "Hope for Treatment of Retired Athletes." www.cyberpt.com/postconcussionpilotstudynfl.asp. Accessed December 1, 2015.

Rossetti, Louis M. *Communication Intervention: Birth to Three*, 2nd ed.. San Diego: Singular Publishing, 2001.

———. *The Rossetti Infant-Toddler Language Scale*. East Moline, IL: LinguaSystems, 2000.

Seigel, Daniel, and Tina Payne Bryson. *The Whole-Brain Child*. New York: Bantam Books, 2011.

Sobsey, Dick. "Marital Stability and Marital Satisfaction in Families of Children with Disabilities: Chicken or Egg?" *Developmental Disabilities Bulletin* 32, no. 1 (2004): 62–83.

Steinman, G., D. Mankuta, R. Zuckerman, and F. Gray, eds. *The Cause of Autism: Concepts and Misconceptions*. New York: Baffin Books, 2014.

Stickler, Kristine R. *Guide to Analysis of Language Transcripts*. Eau Claire, WI: Thinking Publications, 1987.

Swigert, Nancy. "Dysarthria: Understanding and Assessing." Class presented by Linguisystems, Inc, November 2013.

———. "Dysarthria: Practical Approaches to Treatment." Class presented by Linguisystems, Inc. November 2013.

Upledger, John. *A Brain Is Born: Exploring the Birth and Development of the Central Nervous System*. Berkeley, CA: North Atlantic Books. 1996.

———. *CST 1 Study Guide*. Rev. ed. Florida: UI Publishing, 2006.

———. *Pediatrics 1 Study Guide: Skills for Working with Babies, Children and Families*. Rev. ed. Florida: UI Publishing, 2008.

———. *Pediatrics 2 Study Guide*. Rev. ed. Florida: UI Publishing, 2009.

Upledger, John, and Jon Vredevoogd. *Craniosacral Therapy*. Seattle: Eastland Press, 1983.

Vergara, Elise, and Rosemarie Bigsby. *Developmental and Therapeutic Interventions in the NICU*. Baltimore: Paul H. Brookes Publishing, 2004.

Ward, Sally. *Baby Talk: Strengthen Your Child's Ability to Listen, Understand and Communicate*. New York: Ballantine Books, 2001.

Wanveer, Tad. "Autism Spectrum Disorders: How CST Can Help." *Massage Today* 7 (2007): 1–4.

WebMD. Information about sleep disorders. www.webmd.com/sleep-disorders/excessive.sleepiness/10/10-results-sleep-loss. Accessed October 5, 2015.

Williams, Mary Sue, and Sherry Shellenberger. *How Does Your Engine Run? Leader's Guide to the Alert Program for Self-Regulation*. Albuquerque, NM: Therapy Works, 1996.

# INDEX

# ABOUT THE AUTHOR

**Suzanne M. Ducharme**, MS CCC-SLP, is a licensed and ASHA-certified speech language pathologist with over twenty years experience working with children with a range of complex medical and developmental challenges. Suzanne has specialized in working with feeding and swallowing, early language development, and speech disorders. Suzanne is the owner and master clinician of South Shore Speech Pathology Partners, an innovative clinical practice in Weymouth, Massachusetts, that combines traditional SLP services with craniosacral therapy, Reiki, and other alternative healing modalities that support children with special needs and their families. She completed certification in the Holistic Manifestation Method™ of coaching in June 2015 and continues to expand her skills in both speech pathology and alternative therapies. Suzanne has extensive experience in educating and coaching parents, helping them to become better communication partners and advocates for their children. Suzanne has done presentations on the local, state, and national levels covering a range of topics, and she has been active in her professional community, serving as president of the Massachusetts Speech Language Hearing Association from 2007 to 2010 and serving on several ASHA committees. Suzanne recently completed a three-year term as chair of the Board of Licensure for Speech Language Pathology and Audiology in Massachusetts. She lives in Pembroke, Massachusetts, with her partner, Jeff.